CONGENITAL DISORDERS - LABORATORY AND CLINICAL RESEARCH

BICUSPID AORTIC VALVE

DIAGNOSIS, SURGICAL TREATMENT AND COMPLICATIONS

Congenital Disorders - Laboratory and Clinical Research

Additional books in this series can be found on Nova's website under the Series tab.

Additional e-books in this series can be found on Nova's website under the e-book tab.

CONGENITAL DISORDERS - LABORATORY AND CLINICAL RESEARCH

BICUSPID AORTIC VALVE

DIAGNOSIS, SURGICAL TREATMENT AND COMPLICATIONS

ANTHONY CHAPMAN
EDITOR

NOVA BIOMEDICAL

New York

NOTICE TO THE READER

Library of Congress Cataloging-in-Publication Data

ISBN: 978-1-63482-786-7
Library of Congress Control Number: 2015938197

Published by Nova Science Publishers, Inc. † New York

Contents

Preface

Bicuspid aortic valve (BAV) is the most common congenital pathology of the aortic valve occurring in 0.5-2% of the general population and frequently requiring surgical management after the fourth decade of life. From the etiology to the surgical management of BAV is analyzed. Other chapters review genome-wide association studies, linkage analyses and next-generation sequencing studies, which are beginning to build a more comprehensive picture of the genetic bases of BAV. The prospects for developing tools for genetic screening of families and for risk stratification are explored as well, including the future steps which are necessary for the creation of an individualized approach to managing BAV. The last chapter is a review of the present understanding of ascending thoracic aortic aneurysm pathogenesis. The genetic basis and basic pathology underlying BAV and ascending thoracic aortic aneurysms are discussed as well, and are compared to known mechanisms underlying other aortopathologies.

Chapter 1 - Bicuspid aortic valve (BAV) is the most common congenital pathology of the aortic valve, occurring in 0.5-2% of the general population and frequently requiring surgical management after the fourth decade of human life. The natural history of patients with BAV regards the development of aortic valve disease, i.e. aortic stenosis, insufficiency or endocarditis. For these reasons, up to 25% of patients with BAV need for surgical correction. Moreover, the association between BAV and aortic pathology has been described in several studies, such as ascending aorta aneurysm, acute aortic dissection or rupture. Many controversies have been analyzed for a complete clarification of reasons of this association: dilatation of proximal aorta in patients with BAV could be secondary to hemodynamic effects related to flow alterations through abnormal aortic valve or to a primary manifestation of a complex genetic disorder involving both aortic valve and aortic wall. The term "bicuspid aortic valve syndrome" indicates the heterogeneous spectrum of valvular and ascending aorta disease.

Surgical approach to patients with BAV-related aortic disease represents a challenge for cardiac surgeons. The best surgical management and the timing of operation remain unclear, and many studies report different results. Replacement of the valve and/or the aorta can be performed with very low mortality and morbidity, and in the past 20 years valve repair has become an additional option in the presence of mild-to-moderate insufficiency of BAV. Patients with BAV disease are usually younger than patients with degenerative disease affecting a tricuspid aortic valve, and for this reason the optimal treatment is aimed to reach the goal of optimal long-term results in terms of freedom from valve reoperation and complications.

In the author's experience at the Cardiac Surgery Unit of the Tor Vergata University of Rome, BAV disease represents 15-20% of patients operated on for isolated aortic valve replacement. However, this incidence raises up to 35% in presence of ascending aorta dilation requiring surgery.

Different surgical operations have been performed for patients with BAV-related ascending aorta dilatation: in a seven year period, 150 consecutive elective patients (mean age 57.6±13.7 years, 116 males) were treated: 46 patients underwent Bentall operation (Group 1; 31%), 77 (51%) separate aortic valve and ascending aorta replacement and 27 (18%) ascending aorta replacement only with or without BAV repair. Operative mortality was 2.1% (n=1) in Group 1, 1.3% (n=1) in Group 2, and absent in Group 3 (p=NS). The incidence of in-hospital major complications was 4% in Group 1 (n=2), 2.6% in Group 2 (n=2), and absent in Group 3, (p=NS); pacemaker implantation was 4% (n=2), 1.3% (n=1), and absent, respectively (p=NS). At 5 years, survival was 94%±4% for Group 1, 92%±3.4% for Group 2, and 100% for Group 3.

Chapter 2 – Bicuspid Aortic Valve (BAV) is a condition which displays great phenotypic and genotypic variability; a feature which has hindered identification of discrete genetic influences on phenotype. From a genetic perspective, cases range from those associated with known syndromes, such as Turner or Marfan syndromes, to families in whom classic Mendelian patterns of inheritance are observed, to sporadic *de novo* cases with no clear heritability. In addition, the genetic influences on each individual component of the overall BAV phenotype may be separate and complex. In this chapter, the authors review the known syndromes and genetic variants associated with BAV and its complications. They review genome-wide association studies, linkage analyses and next-generation sequencing studies which are beginning to build a more comprehensive picture of the genetic basis of BAV, and will explore how these genetic variants may interact with haemodynamic factors to create an individual phenotype. The authors will also review the prospects for developing tools for genetic screening of families and for risk stratification and explore the future steps which are necessary for creation of an individualised approach to managing BAV.

Chapter 3 – Aortic aneurysms are characterized by weakened aortic walls and are relatively common causes of death because of arterial dissection or rupture. The most common causes of thoracic aortic aneurysm are congenital genetic defects in the aortic wall. These can occur in association with pathological conditions such as Marfan syndrome (MFS) and bicuspid aortic valve (BAV). Many studies have observed similarities between the histology of the aneurysmal tissue of the aorta in MFS and BAV. In MFS, mutations in the gene encoding for the extracellular matrix protein fibrillin-1 have been detected; this mutation leads to dysregulation of transforming growth factor-beta (TGF-b) signaling. In contrast, the genetics underlying BAV are largely unknown. The current grading of aortic abnormalities during histopathological evaluation of BAV is based on conflicting reports. Thus, whether mechanisms related to the existing aneurysmal histological alterations in BAV are due to genetic etiology and/or wall stress induced by flow turbulence requires further investigation. The heritability of BAV is high, estimated at 0.75–0.89. Family-based genome-wide analyses revealed a linkage between BAV and chromosomal regions 5q, 13q, and 18q in autosomal dominant inheritance with reduced penetrance and a non-Mendelian pattern.

A male predominance of more than 3:1 has been reported for BAV, and this anomaly is very frequent in X0 Turner's syndrome (incidence rate: 22–34%), suggesting an X-linked contribution. In one family with Anderson syndrome four family members were described with BAV. In Anderson syndrome, a mutation in the *potassium inwardly-rectifying channel, subfamily J, member 2* is observed. Mutations were detected in the transmembrane receptor *NOTCH1*. Moreover, mutations in the vascular smooth muscle cell alpha actin gene (*ACTA2*) have also been identified in patients with BAV and aortic aneurysms. Furthermore, BAV can manifest as part of defects in the left ventricular outflow tract spectrum including aortic coarctation, arch hypoplasia, and supravalvular and mitral valve stenosis. The *UFD1L* gene, which is highly expressed in the outflow tract during embryogenesis, is down-regulated in the cusps of patients with BAV compared with those of control patients. Heterozygous loss of *Nkx2-5*, *Fgf8*, and *GATA5* in mice predisposes for the development of BAV. Tissue-specific deletion of the gene encoding activin receptor type 1 (*Alk2/Acvr1*) in the cushion mesenchyme is observed to result in formation of aortic valve defects including BAV. Endothelial nitric oxide synthase (eNOS) is also associated with the development of BAV in mice. A high incidence of aortic aneurysms was detected in eNOS/apolipoprotein E double-knockout mice. Recent studies also reported a significant decrease in the amount of the eNOS protein present in aneurysmal BAV aortic tissue compared with tricuspid aortic valve (TAV) tissue. Local differences in eNOS protein expression were observed in BAV compared with TAV aortic aneurysms, probably due to variations in aortic wall shear stresses. Dysregulated TGF-b activity, dysregulation of miRNAs, and loss of aortic medial elastic fibers are observed in ascending aortic aneurysms and acute aortic dissection (AAD). Patients with BAV are at an increased risk of developing AAD (5 to 9 times more than normal; 12.5 to 20.5 times more than patients with MFS).

In this chapter, the authors review the present understanding of ascending thoracic aortic aneurysm pathogenesis. They discuss the genetic basis and basic pathology underlying BAV and ascending thoracic aortic aneurysms, and compare these to known mechanisms underlying other aortopathologies. Histopathological findings in dilated aortic walls of BAV were compared with dilated TAV and MFS.

In: Bicuspid Aortic Valve
Editor: Anthony Chapman
ISBN: 978-1-63482-786-7

Chapter 1

Bicuspid Aortic Valve Syndrome: From the Etiology to the Surgical Strategies of Treatment

Paolo Nardi, MD, PhD*, Marco Russo, MD, Antonio Pellegrino, MD, and Luigi Chiariello, MD

Abstract

Bicuspid aortic valve (BAV) is the most common congenital pathology of the aortic valve, occurring in 0.5-2% of the general population and frequently requiring surgical management after the fourth decade of human life. The natural history of patients with BAV regards the development of aortic valve disease, i.e. aortic stenosis, insufficiency or endocarditis. For these reasons, up to 25% of patients with BAV need for surgical correction. Moreover, the association between BAV and aortic pathology has been described in several studies, such as ascending aorta aneurysm, acute aortic dissection or rupture. Many controversies have been analyzed for a complete clarification of reasons of this association: dilatation of proximal aorta in patients with BAV could be secondary to hemodynamic effects related to flow alterations through abnormal aortic valve or to a primary manifestation of a complex genetic

* Corresponding Author: Paolo Nardi, MD, PhD. Policlinico Universitario Tor Vergata, Tor Vergata University of Rome. Viale Oxford 81. 00133 Rome, Italy. Tel: +39-0620903826. Fax: +39-0620903538. e-mail: pa.nardi4@libero.it

disorder involving both aortic valve and aortic wall. The term "bicuspid aortic valve syndrome" indicates the heterogeneous spectrum of valvular and ascending aorta disease.

Surgical approach to patients with BAV-related aortic disease represents a challenge for cardiac surgeons. The best surgical management and the timing of operation remain unclear, and many studies report different results. Replacement of the valve and/or the aorta can be performed with very low mortality and morbidity, and in the past 20 years valve repair has become an additional option in the presence of mild-to-moderate insufficiency of BAV. Patients with BAV disease are usually younger than patients with degenerative disease affecting a tricuspid aortic valve, and for this reason the optimal treatment is aimed to reach the goal of optimal long-term results in terms of freedom from valve reoperation and complications.

In our experience at the Cardiac Surgery Unit of the Tor Vergata University of Rome, BAV disease represents 15-20% of patients operated on for isolated aortic valve replacement. However, this incidence raises up to 35% in presence of ascending aorta dilation requiring surgery.

Different surgical operations have been performed for patients with BAV-related ascending aorta dilatation: in a seven year period, 150 consecutive elective patients (mean age 57.6±13.7 years, 116 males) were treated: 46 patients underwent Bentall operation (Group 1; 31%), 77 (51%) separate aortic valve and ascending aorta replacement and 27 (18%) ascending aorta replacement only with or without BAV repair. Operative mortality was 2.1% (n=1) in Group 1, 1.3% (n=1) in Group 2, and absent in Group 3 (p=NS). The incidence of in-hospital major complications was 4% in Group 1 (n=2), 2.6% in Group 2 (n=2), and absent in Group 3, (p=NS); pacemaker implantation was 4% (n=2), 1.3% (n=1), and absent, respectively (p=NS). At 5 years, survival was 94%±4% for Group 1, 92%±3.4% for Group 2, and 100% for Group 3.

Bicuspid aortic valve (BAV) is the most common congenital heart defect, with an estimated prevalence in the general population between 0.5% and 2% [1]. Even if in most cases there are no signs of this abnormality lifelong, the altered valvular anatomy represents an important predisposition to the development of both aortic stenosis and insufficiency, or endocarditis. As a result, approximately 25% of patients require valve surgery during their life [2,3]. In addition, BAV is frequently associated with aneurysmal dilatation of the aortic root or ascending thoracic aorta and other diseases, such as aortic dissection and aortic coarctation [4]. These associations are likely related to a genetic disorder. At the same time, much evidence shows that hemodynamic alterations and flow patterns through the anatomically altered aortic valve seem to be able to determine an incremented shear stress on the aortic wall that could induce degeneration of the elastic fibers of the tunica media, finally resulting in the dilatation of the aortic vessel [5]. The interaction between genetic predisposition and hemodynamic factors probably constitute the pathogenesis for the development of the disease [6]. Therefore, the scenario of BAV syndrome seems to be very complex and the complete comprehension of pathophysiology, clinical implications and optimal treatment, especially for patients affected by valve disease and aortic dilation remain still unclear.

Definition and Epidemiology of Aortic Pathology

The relationship between BAV and congenital and acquired diseases of the thoracic aorta, such as aortic coarctation, ectasia and aneurysm of the ascending aorta and acute dissection, has been extensively documented in Literature [5].

In particular, the tendency to develop ascending aorta aneurysm (Figure 1) and acute aortic complications has also been described also in the absence of significant alterations of BAV [7].

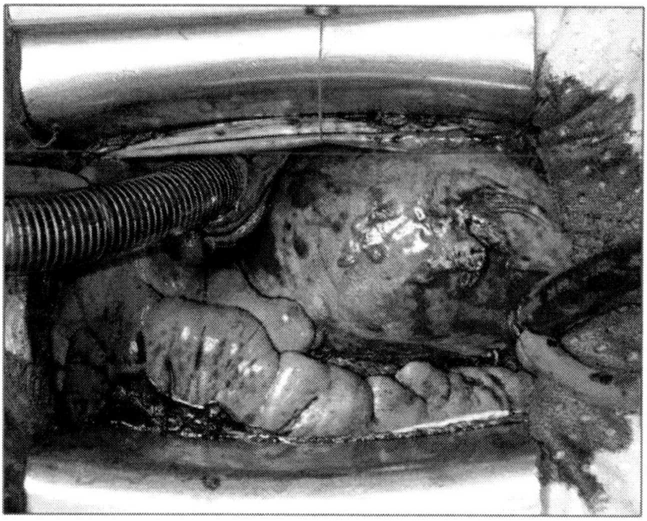

Figure 1. Ascending aorta aneurysm in a patient with BAV (intraoperative view).

At this regard, it has been recently introduced the term "bicuspid aortic valve (BAV) syndrome", indicating the heterogeneous spectrum of valvular and aortic disease in presence of BAV [8].

From the epidemiological point of view, frequency of aortic dilatation in patients with BAV is differently estimated and this depends on the criteria used to define the dilatation and the studied populations. In the largest series (i.e. Olmsted Country Series) it has been reported an initial prevalence of 15% which increased up to 39% at the end of the study [2]. Other series reported percentages ranging between 35% and 80% [9]. Recently, Michelena and Co-workers have reported a risk for the development of an ascending aorta aneurysm of the 26% at 25 years, with an incidence of 84.9 /10.000 patient-years that appeared significantly higher in comparison to that observed in the general population [10].

Sex, age, hypertension, functional status of the aortic valve are important risk factors for aortic dilatation [1]. Different risk factors have been proposed for the dilation of aortic root and ascending aorta. Male sex, age over 60 years, and severe aortic regurgitation are predictors of disease in the first portion of the aorta, while age between 50 and 60 years, high blood pressure and severe valvular stenosis are associated with the expansion of the ascending aorta at the supracoronary level, so involving in 79% of cases ascending thoracic aorta and in 58% the aortic root also [9].

Acute aortic dissection (Figure 2) is 5-10 times more common in patients with BAV in comparison with patients with tricuspid aortic valve, even in the absence of hypertension, coarctation of the aorta or valvular disease. Recently, the incidence of aortic dissection in BAV patients has been defined as 3.1 /10.000 patients-year, with an adjusted risk for the age about 8 times higher than in the general population. This disease usually affects younger patients, presenting about ten years before than in those with tricuspid valve [10]. Aortic dimensions are a major risk factor for acute aortic dissection, but have a limited role in predicting the acute aortic syndrome, because many events occur in patients with a normal aortic diameter [11]. Male sex, family history, Turner's syndrome, coarctation of the aorta and aortic wall stiffness are risk factors equally important for the development of acute dissection [12].

Family history of BAV has an important role: about 32% of first degree relatives of people with BAV have a dilatation of the aortic root with a significant reduction in the elasticity and increased stiffness of the wall, as showed by echocardiographic studies [13].

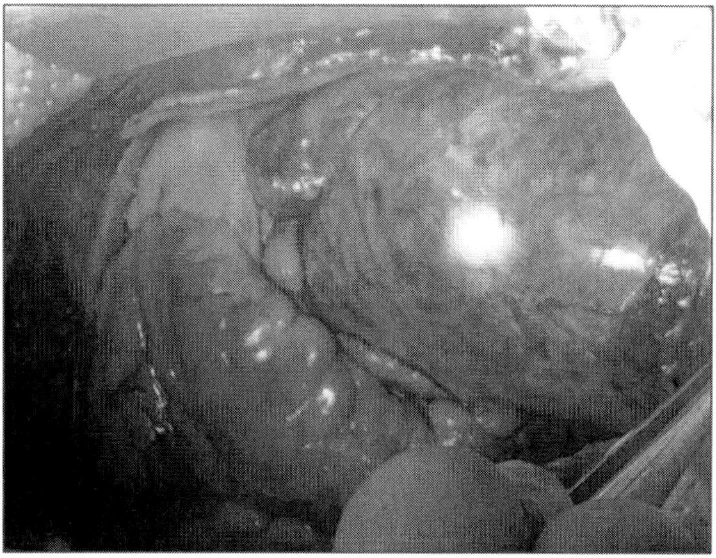

Figure 2. Acute aortic dissection in a patient with BAV (operative view).

Etiopathogenesis of the Aortic Disease

The disease of the aorta associated with BAV recognizes a multiple and complex pathogenesis. Historically, strictly hemodynamic factors have been proposed to describe the dilatation of the ascending aorta as post-stenotic compared to a valvular orifice congenitally altered [6]. The problem is certainly much more complex, and several levels of evidence, with data often conflicting, led to the formulation of two major theories: the first, purely genetic, interprets the presence of BAV as a complex set of molecular and gene expression alterations affecting both the valve and the first portion of the aorta that makes tissues more prone to dilation; the second one interprets the complex hemodynamic alterations and flow patterns through the BAV as main stressors for the aortic wall, capable to induce a tissue remodeling that gradually leads to a reduction of the elasticity of the vessel, and then progressively to dilation [14]. The dilation of the aortic root and ascending aorta has been documented also during childhood [15].

The genetic theory has become very popular in recent decades, and has framed BAV as a complex congenital disorder of connective tissue. The presence of BAV is associated with dilatation of the ascending thoracic aorta more frequently than in patients with tricuspid valve [6], also in those patients with a normally functioning aortic valve, thereby indicating the presence of an intrinsic major susceptibility of the aortic wall to progressive dilation [15]. In addition, studying the first-degree relatives of people with BAV, there is a prevalence of aortic dilation of 32%, with a statistically significant difference compared to a control group of patients with tricuspid valve and no any relative affected. The same study also characterized the aortic wall in terms of elasticity and rigidity, describing intermediate characteristics between patients with BAV, their first-degree relatives with tricuspid valve and the control group, suggesting how fundamental is the intrinsic genetically predisposition to the development of aortic dilatation and describing the first-degree relatives as an intermediate phenotype between those with tricuspid valve and those presenting BAV [13].

Very interesting data are reported in retrospective studies that have analyzed the fate of the ascending aorta in patients undergoing aortic valve replacement with intraoperative finding of bicuspid valve. Russo and Co-workers described in a group of 50 patients followed during 19±3.9 years: they reported 10% rate of acute aortic rupture/dissection, 15% rate of sudden death and 6% rate of reoperation on the ascending aorta, with a cumulative event rate of 30% [16].

Goland et al. described a cumulative rate of 4.8% of aortic events with no aortic dissection and a just single reoperation in a database of 252 patients with BAV (median follow-up 8.9±6.3 years) [17]. A maximum transverse diameter of 45 mm at the time of aortic valve replacement has been identified as a predictor of future aortic complications. For these reasons, current guidelines suggest this value as a cut of for ascending aorta replacement during aortic valve replacement [18].

One of the main arguments in favor of the genetic theory was based on histological findings of cystic degeneration of the media in the aorta of patients with BAV and those affected by Marfan Syndrome. Recent molecular investigations have shown important differences in the pattern of extracellular matrix protein architecture in the two diseases, highlighting an asymmetric distribution of tissue alterations in BAV aorta, probably due to a tissue remodeling induced by an abnormal wall stress [14].

The presence of dilatation of the pulmonary artery, as well intracranial aneurysms and an increased risk of spontaneous dissections of neck vessels in patients with BAV suggest for a major genetically determined predisposition for the development of aneurysms [7].

The hemodynamic theory was formulated by Robicsek and Colleagues, who have experimentally demonstrated that a functionally normal BAV is morphologically stenotic and produces a turbulent and eccentric transvalvular flow determining an asymmetric wall stress on the ascending aorta [19]. This concept was supported by in vivo data from studies based on nuclear magnetic resonance, according to which the different morphologies of BAV differently contribute to the genesis of systolic helical and swirling flows. Thus, the most common variant of the BAV, with the fusion of the right and left coronary cusps, produces a systolic jet directed anterior and to the right, with the involvement of the aortic root and the great convexity of ascending aorta. On the other hand, the latero-lateral subtype is associated with a jet directed posteriorly and to the left, with a predominant involvement of the proximal portion of the aortic arch [20]. These differences had already been highlighted in clinical setting [21]. Normally, through the normal aortic valve we observe a systolic flow swirling limited to the sinuses of Valsalva and involved in the correct diastolic coronary perfusion. In the BAV the helical flows extend to other portions of the proximal aorta resulting in a significant increase in local wall stress. The jet with high speed and turbulence, impacting on the aortic wall, would determine therefore a remodeling of the same, consisting in the activation of extracellular matrix degradation, due to the activation of metalloproteinase-2 and -9. There is also an associated deficiency of fibrillin-1 [22] and the apoptosis in smooth muscle cells through the expression of specific proteins that contribute to the impairment of the aortic wall. Such mechanisms would then lead to a local degradation of collagen and elastin with increasing of the distance between elastic fibers, cellular atrophy and architectural disorganization of smooth muscle cells, determining a greater parietal fragility and a reduced elasticity. These changes would be responsible for the progressive and localized aneurismal dilatation of the aorta and could explain why in patients with BAV-related ascending aorta disease there is a typical asymmetry of aneurysm, mainly involving the great convexity [14].

Although seemingly in contrast, the two most popular theories are not mutually exclusive: in presence of a molecular-genetic substrate not yet totally described, hemodynamic factors, potentially increased by further modification of the physiology of the cusps, could act by triggering histological and structural changes on an aorta already predisposed, thus determining disease progression. Moreover, the two factors could contribute in different ways depending on the section of the aorta affected by the aneurismal dilation. Most likely, therefore, the complexity of BAV-related aortic disease can be explained according to the hypothesis of a multifactorial etiology, in which genetic and acquired factors contribute together [6].

Histology of the Aortic Wall

Many studies have demonstrated the presence of specific histological changes in the aortic wall of patients with BAV. In particular, degeneration of the extracellular matrix, cystic necrosis, fragmentation of elastic fibers with increase of their distance and elastic atrophy, increase the expression of metalloproteinases and reduce the inhibitors of the same. These changes can be associated with the risk of aortic rupture and/or dissection. It is very important to stress that 45% of patients with aortic diameters considered normal, because less than 45 mm, present already high degree of histological alterations. Larson and Edwards have defined an histopathological classification system in 5 degrees [23]:

I. Absence of injury
II. Lesions involving 1-10% of the arterial tunica media
III. Lesions involving 11-25% of the arterial tunica media
IV. Lesions involving 26-50% of the arterial tunica media
V. Injuries involving 51-100% of the arterial tunica media

Anatomic Classification and Natural History

Disease of the aorta in patients with BAV is expressed in a heterogeneous mix of different phenotypic variants that probably recognize different pathogenic influences.

The determination of the *aortic ratio* according to the Roman formula is fundamental to define the characteristics of the aneurysm. A ratio of 1.1 is used to define a dilated aorta in respect to the body surface area and age and a value of 1.4 indicates a serious dilatation [24].

The most common condition appears to be the expansion of the tubular tract of ascending aorta over sino-tubular junction with a normal or just moderately dilated aortic root. This phenotype affects approximately 70% of patients, most females and mainly associated with aortic valve stenosis. The age, with a maximum risk between 50 and 60 years, and high blood pressure are independent predictors of this phenomenon.

The dilation of the aortic root with the tubular tract of the ascending aorta moderately dilated or normally preserved, interests about 13% of patients, who are usually males, younger and are affected by aortic regurgitation.

Different phenotypes of bicuspid valve have been associated with different patterns of aortic aneurysm: the antero-posterior variant is associated more frequently with dilatation of the aortic root or ascending aorta, while the latero-lateral variant is more associated with ascending aorta aneurysm with involvement of the proximal portion of the aortic arch. An aorta of normal diameter, with aortic ratio between 0.9 and 1.1, seems to be more rare than the two previous phenotypes (11%) and is typically present in younger patients, in which the aging factor have not yet enough impact.

It has been described, finally, a last phenotype called *small aorta* with an aortic diameter ratio less than 0.9 or a maximum aortic diameter less than 29 mm. This variant affects approximately 6% of the population and it is usually associated with significant degrees of aortic valve stenosis and mitral valve regurgitation. This small group of patients represents certainly an anomaly as compared to the general trend, and reflects a general disorder of vessel embryology [9].

The incidence of aortic rupture or dissection is 3.1 /10.000 patient-year and seems to be about eight times more common in BAV patients than in those with tricuspid aortic valve [10].

The rate of aortic diameter expansion is greater in BAV as compared with tricuspid valve (.19 versus .13 cm/year). The role of aortic valve stenosis as predictor of rapid progression and aortic complications has been shown in a study of 514 cases of aneurysms of the ascending aorta not operated [25]. In relation to the risk of an acute aortic syndrome, currently international guidelines recommend a more aggressive surgical treatment, indicating surgery at a maximum transverse diameter between 45 and 50 mm in patients with BAV. If the patients need aortic valve surgery a diameter of the ascending aorta greater than 45 mm should be an indication at the same time. Many Authors have argued for the need, especially in young patients, to perform a prophylactic replacement of the ascending aorta regardless of its size, but there are not convincing data on this regard [26].

Diagnosis

Echocardiographic assessment is the gold standard for the diagnostic management of patients with BAV. The evaluation should include a complete visualization of aortic annulus, root, sino-tubular junction and distal segments of the ascending aorta since the aortic arch. In the parasternal long-axis view, the size of the aortic root can be measured perpendicular to the longitudinal axis of the aortic lumen at four levels: 1) the annulus, which is measured at the hinge point of the cusps method with inner-to-inner; 2) sinuses of Valsalva; 3) sino-tubular junction; 4) ascending aorta with a method leading-to-leading (Figure 3) [27].

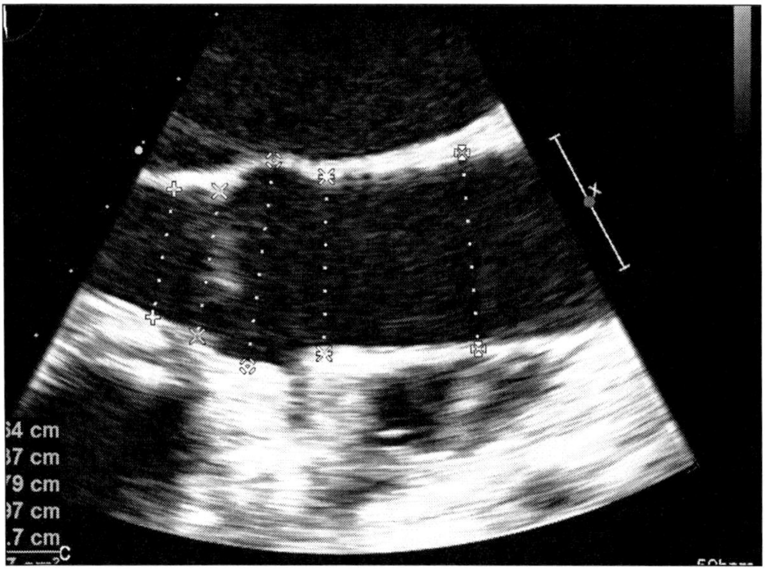

Figure 3. Echocardiographic assessment of aortic root and ascending aorta.

All the measures should be taken during the end of the diastole. The measurement of the annulus seems to be crucial because diameter seems to well correlate with the presence of histopathological changes in the arterial media of the aortic root and of the ascending aorta, regardless of their size. The evaluation of the aortic arch can be performed with trans-jugular approach.

In the evaluation of the patient during the progression of the disease is necessary, when we make a comparison between the various examinations, taking into account the measurement technique used in relation to the various phases of the cardiac cycle, the landmarks and the measurement mode, consisting in "inclusion" or "non-inclusion" of the aortic wall in the measurement.

In patients with poor visualization of all segments of aorta when maximum transverse diameter is greater than 40 mm computed tomography and/or magnetic resonance of the whole aorta is strongly recommended (Figure 4).

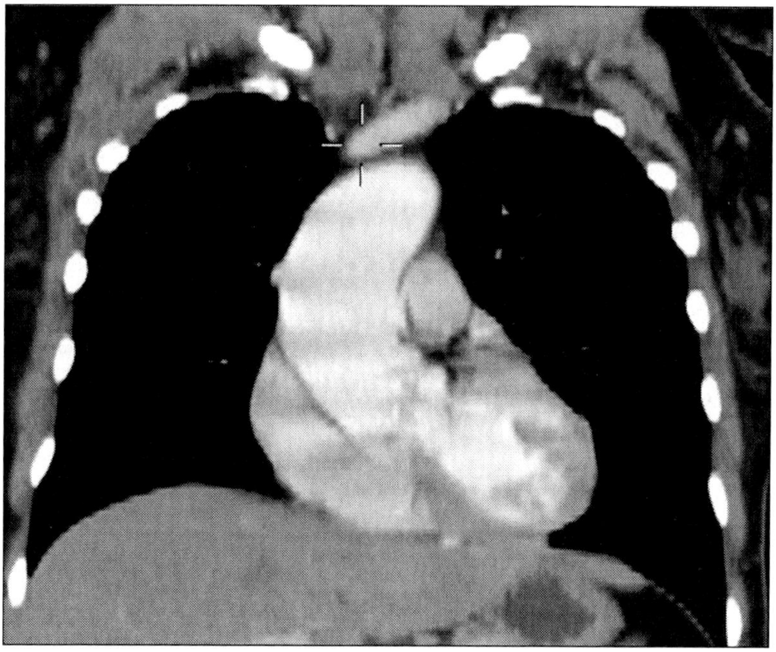

Figure 4. CT-scan of aorta showing ascending aorta dilation in patient affected by BAV syndrome (MP reconstruction).

Acute aortic dissection clinically appears with sudden and migrant chest pain and it could be often associated with signs of cardiogenic shock, hypotension, cerebral or peripheral ischemic complications. Taking into account a diagnostic doubt and analyze the possible differential diagnosis such as myocardial infarction, pulmonary embolism, pneumothorax and rupture of the stomach, it is fundamental for a correct clinical management of these patients the execution of an emergency computerized tomography with contrast medium, in order to display the possible flap dissection, the extent of the dissection itself or the presence of site of rupture is of crucial importance. This diagnostic tool appears with high diagnostic sensitivity (96%) and specificity (98%), is characterized by a rapid execution speed, and it is possible a multi-slice spiral acquisition (Figure 5).

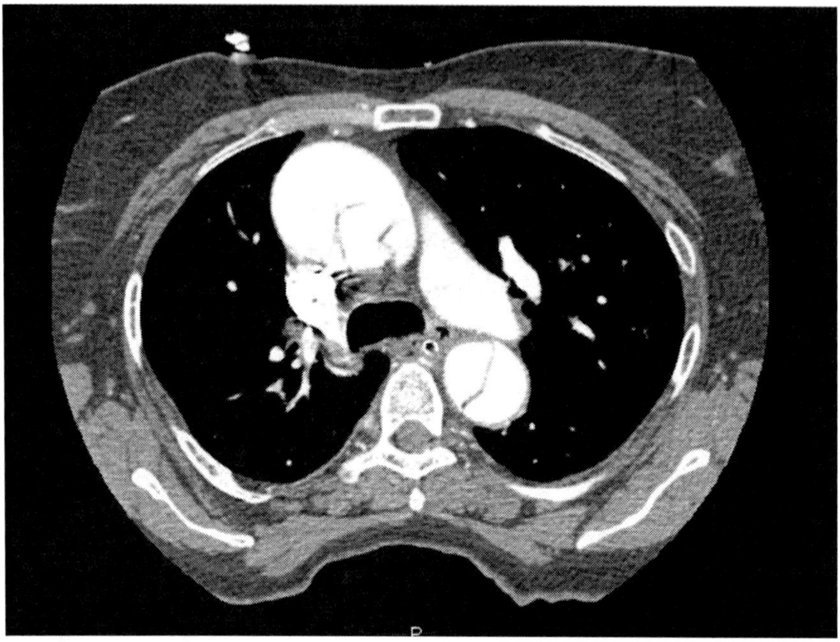

Figure 5. CT-scan with contrast medium showing a flap of dissection in the mild part of ascending aorta.

Surgical Treatment

The incidence of BAV in isolated aortic valve replacement ranges approximately at 15-20% of cases, while, in presence of aortic dilation, up to 35%.

Indication for surgical treatment of aortic root and ascending aorta in patients with BAV is more aggressive respect to tricuspid aortic valve patients mainly due to a greater incidence of acute aortic complications observed during the follow-up of these patients [28]. Isolated replacement of the aortic root or ascending aorta is recommended for diameters of the aorta at 45-50 mm. According with the general opinion regarding the intrinsic predisposition to dilation of the aortic wall in BAV patients, the cut-off beyond which there is surgical indication is shifted down by 50 mm as compared to patients with tricuspid valve. Need for aortic valve replacement changes further the cut-off for surgery. If the patients undergoes aortic valve replacement ascending aorta should be treated when diameter is > 45 mm. Moreover, in presence of a documented rapid growth of aortic dimensions, with value greater than 5 mm

/year or in cases of Turner's syndrome, surgical treatment can be considered even for smaller diameters. It should be take into account also the opportunity to index the aortic dimensions to the body surface area preoperatively. An aortic ratio > 1.4 represents the cut-off above which surgical replacement of the aorta is strongly recommended [29].

Planning of the surgical strategy depends on the characteristics of the patient, the age, the presence of a relevant valve disease [30-31].

Treatment of dilated ascending aorta with a normally functioning BAV, depends on the anatomy of the aneurysm and the involvement of the aortic root. In particular, if the latter is not interested, it is possible a supra-coronary ascending aorta replacement only, using a vascular tubular Dacron prosthesis, anastomosing the proximal part of the prosthesis to the sino-tubular junction and distally to the proximal portion of the aortic arch. The reconstruction of the sino-tubular junction can restore the competence of the aortic valve in presence of a moderate insufficiency secondarily determined by an excessive commissural stretching [32].

Moreover, if a major alteration of valve cusps is not present, good results can be obtained with the replacing the aortic root using the valve-sparing techniques, preserving the native valve and re-implanting it in a vascular graft according to the David procedure, or remodeling the aortic root according to the Yacoub procedure. Both techniques require the re-implantation of the coronary ostia on the tubular graft prosthesis. David operation seems to provide excellent results in BAV patients. El Khoury has reported a 100% freedom from reoperation and moderate-to-severe aortic regurgitation in a six-year follow-up period [33].

When both aorta and aortic valve are diseased surgical approach depends on the anatomy of the aortic root. If the aortic root is preserved we can replace the valve and ascending aorta separately. If the aortic root is dilated (diameter > 45 mm) and BAV is affected by a primary disease (insufficiency or mixed pathology) Bentall-DeBono operation guarantees optimal. The operation consists on the entire replacement of the aortic root and ascending aorta using a composite valved conduit graft with the re-implantation of the coronary ostia on the tubular graft [34]. Etz and Co-workers analyzed data from 206 BAV patients subjected to Bentall operation during a 18-year period. During a mean follow-up of 5.9 years no patient required reoperation on the ascending aorta. Long-term survival was 93% after 5 years and 89% after 10 years, respectively, and survival estimate was equivalent to that observed in the normal age- and sex-matched population [35].

Our Experience

We reported data on BAV and ascending aortic surgery performed during a 7-year period (2005-2011) at the Cardiac Surgery Unit of the Tor Vergata University of Rome [31]. One-hundred and fifty consecutive elective patients affected by ascending aorta aneurysm and BAV (mean age 57.6±13.7 years, 116 males, 77%) underwent surgery. Bentall operation was performed in 46 patients (31%, Group 1), separate aortic valve and ascending aorta replacement in 77 (51%, Group 2), ascending aorta replacement only with or without BAV repair in 27 (18%, Group 3). This population of patients represented 30% of all the ascending aortic replacement procedures (n=497), either involving or not the aortic root, electively performed at the same time at our Institution.

Surgical indication to perform Bentall procedure was given in presence of both aortic root and ascending aorta diameter ≥ 45 mm in association with a diseased BAV (severe aortic stenosis in 17 cases, moderate or severe aortic regurgitation in the other cases); to perform separate aortic valve and ascending aorta replacement in presence of a dilated ascending aorta (diameter > 45 mm) and a non-dilated or mildly dilated aortic root (diameter < 45 mm) and of a diseased BAV (moderate or severe aortic stenosis in 52 patients, mixed pathology in the other cases); to perform ascending aorta replacement only with or without BAV repair in presence of a dilation of the supra-coronary proximal ascending aorta > 45 mm, with normal or near-to-normal aortic root and in presence of a non-calcified, normally functioning or less than mildly regurgitating aortic valve.

Operative mortality included death in hospital after operation or within 30 days after discharge. Mean duration of follow-up was 50±23 months. Follow-up was 97% complete. Follow-up echocardiographic data were analyzed and compared with those recorded during in-hospital stay.

As compared with Group 2 and 3, patients in Group 1 were younger, with a higher grade of aortic regurgitation, lower left ventricular ejection fraction, greater left ventricular end-diastolic and end-systolic diameters ($p<0.05$, for all comparisons). As compared with Group 1 ad Group 3, Group 2 patients presented a higher value of 1000arterial pulmonary pressure ($p<0.05$, for both comparisons). Moderate or severe aortic stenosis was detected in 17 paticnts of Group 1 (37%), in 52 of Group 2 (68%) and in no patient of Group 3 ($p\leq0.001$, for all comparisons).

Extracorporeal circulation and aortic cross-clamp times were significantly shorter for Group 3 vs. Group 1 and 2, and shorter for Group 2 in comparison with Group 1 ($p<0.01$, for all comparisons).

Operative mortality was 2.1% (n=1) in Group 1, 1.3% (n=1) in Group 2, absent in Group 3 (p=NS). The incidence of in-hospital major complications was 4% in Group 1 (n=2), 2.6% in Group 2 (n=2), absent in Group 3, (p=NS); need of pacemaker implantation was 4% (n=2), 1.3% (n=1), and absent, respectively (p=NS).

At 5 years, survival was 94%±4% for Group 1, 92%±3.4% for Group 2, 100% for Group 3 (p=NS). Incidence of late death, valve prosthesis-related complications, and need of pacemaker implantation in each group of patients is reported in Table 1.

Table 1. Late Complications

Events	Group 1	Group 2	Group 3	*P*
Death (%)	7	6.8	0	NS
Complications prosthesis-related (%)	7	4.1	0	NS
Permanent pacemaker implantation (%)	4.6	5.5	0	NS

NS = not significant.

Predictor of late death was the advanced age at operation (69±9 years vs. 58±15 years; $p<0.05$). No late complications in any Group related to proximal aorta surgical procedure were recorded during the follow-up period, so no patient required a reoperation on the proximal ascending aorta.

Follow-up echocardiography showed a statistically significant improvement of the left ventricular ejection fraction in patients subjected to Bentall procedure (from 0.56 ± 0.09 preoperatively to 0.60 ± 0.09 during follow-up, $p<0.05$). In Group 2 and 3 was observed no increase in the dimensions of the native aortic root. Moreover, in these two groups of patients, the aortic root diameters were significantly smaller than the preoperative diameters. In Group 2 the size of the root remained stable in all examined patients and an increase of the root diameter greater than 2 mm was not observed in any case. In 1 patient of Group 3 (3.8%) the size of the root increased from 43 mm preoperatively to 46 mm. The mean value of aortic regurgitation grade in patients in which the BAV was repaired or spared did not increase during follow-up (0.5±0.8 /4+) in comparison with the preoperative value (0.8±0.9 /4+). NYHA class of patients is reported in Table 2.

Table 2. Clinical condition during follow-up

	Group 1	Group 2	Group 3	*P*
NYHA class (mean value)	1.0±0.3*	1.1±0.5*	1.1±0.2*	NS

**P*<0.01 vs. preoperative values.
NYHA = New York heart Association.
NS = not significant.

Discussion

Bicuspid aortic valve complications include aortic valve regurgitation, stenosis or a combination of both, and also a greater risk of valve endocarditis [36-38]. In the last years, it has been observed that patients with BAV are predisposed to development of aortic root and ascending aorta dilation, which may lead to dissection or rupture of the aorta even in absence of BAV dysfunction. Furthermore, ascending aortic dilation can progress even after aortic valve replacement [39-43]. For these reasons, a more aggressive surgical treatment even of a moderately enlarged aorta has been recently advocated [44-45]. Depending on the involvement of ascending aorta with or without root dilation and the function of BAV, several more conservative techniques can be adopted. In fact, although the progressive dilation of the ascending aorta is well documented in presence of BAV, the risk of progressive enlargement of the Valsalva sinuses after surgery is less clear [46-47]. This issue has a practical significance, because composite root replacement (i.e. Bentall procedure) requires re-implantation of the coronary ostia, thus resulting in a more demanding procedure carrying an incremental surgical risk as compared to isolated ascending aorta replacement or to separate replacement of aorta and aortic valve [48-49].

In presence of a normally functioning BAV, repair techniques of the aortic valve may prove to be effective in the long term, avoiding valve prostheses-related complications or the need of lifelong anticoagulation therapy [50-52]. Our study seems to confirm that BAV pathology includes a heterogeneous group of patients in which three different surgical strategies may confer satisfactory early and follow-up results when the indication of each type of procedure is carefully done.

In younger patients with aggressive BAV pathology (i.e. aortic root dilation > 45 mm and significant aortic valve regurgitation or dysfunction) Bentall operation confirms as the gold standard therapy [35], and improving of left ventricular function has been showed by means of this surgical technique, even in presence of preoperative advanced aortic insufficiency and left ventricular dysfunction.

In presence of a less pronounced dilation of the root, separate aortic valve and ascending aorta replacement represents a simpler procedure that can be more appropriate especially in presence of older patients.

Isolated ascending aorta replacement represents a safe alternative in presence of normal or near to normal functioning BAV at the time of operation, and the risk of valve dysfunction, at least in a mid-term follow-up period, seems to be negligible.

References

[1] Siu SC, Silversides CK. Bicuspid aortic valve disease. *J Am Coll Cardiol* 2010;55:2789-800.

[2] Michelena HI, Desjardins VA, Avierinos JF, et al. Natural history of asymptomatic patients with normally functioning or minimally dysfunctional bicuspid aortic valve in the community. *Circulation* 2008;117:2776-84.

[3] Ward C. Clinical significance of the bicuspid aortic valve. *Heart* 2000;83:81-5.

[4] Cecconi M, Nistri S, Quarti A, et al. Aortic dilatation in patients with bicuspid aortic valve. *J Cardiovasc Med* 2006;7:11-20.

[5] Braveman AC. Aortic involvement in patients with bicuspid aortic valve. Heart 2011;97:506-13.

[6] Girdauskas E, Borger MA, Secknus MA, Girdauskas G, Kuntze T. Is aortopathy in bicuspid aortic valve disease a congenital defect or a result of abnormal hemodynamics? A critical reappraisal of a one-sided argument. *Eur J Cardiothorac Surg* 2011;39:809-14.

[7] Nistri S, Basso C, Thiene G. Bicuspid aortic valve. *G Ital Cardiol* 2012;13:25-37.

[8] Sorrell VL, Pancyzk E, Alpert JS. A new disease: bicuspid aortic valve aortopathy syndrome. *Am J Med* 2012;125:322-3.

[9] Della Corte A, Bancone C, Quarto C, et al. Predictors of ascending aortic dilatation with bicuspid aortic valve: a wide spectrum of disease expression. *Eur J Cardiothorac Surg* 2007;31:397-404.

[10] Michelena HI, Khanna AD, Mahoney D, et al. Incidence of aortic complications in patients with bicuspid aortic valves. *JAMA* 2011;306:1104-12.

[11] Pape LA, Tsai TT, Isselbacher EM, et al. International Registry of Acute Aortic Dissection (IRAD) Investigators. Aortic diameter > or = 5.5 cm is not a good predictor of type A aortic dissection: observations from the International Registry of Acute Aortic Dissection (IRAD). *Circulation* 2007;116:1120-7.

[12] Nistri S, Grande-Allen J, Noale M, et al. Aortic elasticity and size in bicuspid aortic valve syndrome. *Eur Heart J* 2008;29:472-9.

[13] Biner S, Rafique AM, Ray I, Cuk O, Siegel RJ, Tolstrup K. Aortopathy is prevalent in relatives of bicuspid aortic valve patients. *J Am Coll Cardiol* 2009;53:2288-95.

[14] Della Corte A, De Santo LS, Montagnani S, et al. Spatial patterns of matrix protein expression in dilated ascending aorta with aortic regurgitation: congenital bicuspid valve versus Marfan's syndrome. *J Heart Valve Dis* 2006;15:20-7.

[15] Beroukhim RS, Kruzick TL, Taylor AL, Gao D, Yetman AT. Progression of aortic dilation in children with a functionally normal bicuspid aortic valve. *Am J Cardiol* 2006;98:828-30.

[16] 1000Russo CF, Mazzetti S, Garatti A, et al. Aortic complications after bicuspid aortic valve replacement: long-term results. *Ann Thorac Surg* 2002;74:S1773-6.

[17] Goland S, Czer LS, De Robertis MA, et al. Risk factors associated with reoperation and mortality in 252 patients after aortic valve replacement for congenitally bicuspid aortic valve disease. *Ann Thorac Surg* 2007;83:931-7.

[18] Borger MA, Preston M, Ivanov J, et al. Should the ascending aorta be replaced more frequently in patients with bicuspid aortic valve disease? *J Thorac Cardiovasc Surg* 2004;128:677-83.

[19] Robicsek F, Thbrikar ML, Cook JW, Fowler B. The congenitally bicuspid aortic valve: how does it function? Why does it fail? Ann Thorac Surg 2004;77:177-85.

[20] Hope MD, Hope TA, Meadows AK, et al. Bicuspid aortic valve: four-dimensional MR evaluation of ascending aortic systolic flow patterns. *Radiology* 2010;255:53-61.

[21] Fazel SS, Mallidi HR, Lee RS, et al. The aortopathy of bicuspid aortic valve disease has distinctive patterns and usually involves the transverse aortic arch. *J Thorac Cardiovasc Surg* 2008;135:901-7.

[22] 10003Fedak PW, de Sa MP, Verma S, et al. Vascular matrix remodeling in patients with bicuspid aortic valve malformations: implications for aortic dilatation. *J Thorac Cardiovasc Surg* 2003;126:797-806.

[23] Leone O, Biagini E, Pacini D, et al. The elusive link between aortic wall histology and echocardiographic anatomy in bicuspid aortic valve: implications for prophylactic surgery. *Eur J Cardiothorac Surg* 2012;41:322-7.

[24] Roman MJ, Devereux RB, Niles NW, et al. Aortic root dilatation as a cause of isolated, severe aortic regurgitation. Prevalence, clinical and echocardiographic patterns, and relation to left ventricular hypertrophy and function. *Ann Intern Med* 1987;106:800-7.

[25] Davies RR, Kaple RK, Mandapati D, et al. Natural history of ascending aortic aneurysms in the setting of an unreplaced bicuspid aortic valve. *Ann Thorac Surg* 2007;83:1338-44.

[26] Sundt TM. Replacement of the ascending aorta in bicuspid aortic valve disease: where do we draw the line? *J Thorac Cardiovasc Surg* 2010;140:S41-4.

[27] Evangelista A, Flachskampf FA, Erbel R, et al. Echocardiography in aortic diseases: EAE recommendations for clinical practice. *Eur J Echocardiogr* 2010;11:645-58.

[28] Park CB, Greason KL, Suri RM, Michelena HI, Schaff HV, Sundt TM. Should the proximal arch be routinely replaced in patients with bicuspid aortic valve disease and ascending aortic aneurysm? *J Thorac Cardiovasc Surg* 2011;142:602-7.

[29] Bonow RO, Carabello BA, Chatterjee K, et al. 2008 focused update incorporated into the ACC/AHA 2006 guidelines for the management of patients with valvular heart disease: a report of the American College of Cardiology/American Heart Association Task Force on Practice Guidelines (Writing Committee to revise the 1998 guidelines for the management of patients with valvular heart disease). Endorsed by the Society of Cardiovascular Anesthesiologists, Society for Cardiovascular Angiography and Interventions, and Society of Thoracic Surgeons. *J Am Coll Cardiol* 2008;52:e1-e142.

[30] Della Corte A, Body SC, Booher AM, et al. The International Bicuspid Aortic Valve Consortium (BAVCon) Investigators. Surgical treatment of bicuspid aortic valve disease: Knowledge gaps and research perspectives. *J Thorac Cardiovasc Surg* 2014;147:1749-57.

[31] Nardi P, Pellegrino A, Russo M, Saitto G, Bertoldo F, Chiariello L. Midterm Results of Different Surgical Techniques to Replace Dilated

Ascending Aorta Associated With Bicuspid Aortic Valve Disease. *Ann Thorac Surg* 2013;96:1648-55.

[32] Borger MA, David TE. Management of the valve and ascending aorta in adults with bicuspid aortic valve disease. *Semin Thorac Cardiovasc Surg* 2005;17:143-7.

[33] de Kerchove L, Boodhwani M, Glineur D, et al. Valve sparing-root replacement with the reimplantation technique to increase the durability of bicuspid aortic valve repair. *J Thorac Cardiovasc Surg* 2011;142:1430-8.

[34] Bentall H, De Bono A. A technique for complete replacement of the ascending aorta. *Thorax* 1968;23:338-9.

[35] Etz CD, Homann TM, Silovitz D, et al. Long-term survival after the Bentall procedure in 206 patients with bicuspid aortic valve. *Ann Thorac Surg* 2007;84:1186-94.

[36] Tutar E, Ekici F, Atalay S, Nacar N. The prevalence of bicuspid aortic valve in newborns by echocardiographic screening. *Am Heart J* 2005;150:513-5.

[37] Braverman AC, Güven H, Beardslee MA, Makan M, Kates AM, Moon MR. The bicuspid aortic valve. *Curr Probl Cardiol* 2005;30:470-522.

[38] Nistri S, Basso C, Marzari C, Mormino P, Thiene G. Frequency of bicuspid aortic valve in young male conscripts by echocardiogram. *Am*

[39] *1000charrsid10356185 J Cardiol* 2005;96:718-21.

[40] Michelena HI, Khanna AD, Mahoney D, et al. Incidence of aortic complications in patients with bicuspid aortic valves. *JAMA* 2011;306:1104-12.

[41] Sareyyupoglu B, Suri RM, Schaff HV, et al. Survival and reoperation risk following bicuspid aortic valve-sparing root replacement. *J Heart Valve Dis* 2009;18:1-8.

[42] Davies RR, Kaple RK, Mandapati D, et al. Natural history of ascending aortic aneurysms in the setting of an unreplaced bicuspid aortic valve. *Ann Thorac Surg* 2007;83:1338-44.

[43] Russo CF, Cannata A, Lanfranconi M, Vitali E, Garatti A, Bonacina E. Is aortic wall degeneration related to bicuspid aortic valve anatomy in patients with valvular disease? *J Thorac Cardiovasc Surg* 2008;136:937-42.

[44] Roberts WC, Vowels TJ, Ko JM, et al. Comparison of the structure of the aortic valve and ascending aorta in adults having aortic valve replacement for aortic stenosis versus for pure aortic regurgitation and

resection of the ascending aorta for aneurysm. *Circulation* 2011;123:896-903.

[45] Bassano C, Fratticci L, Del Giudice C, et al. Ectasia of the ascending aorta at the time of aortic valve surgery: replace or relax? *Ital Heart J* 2005;6:968-71.

[46] Hiratzka LF, Bakris GL, Beckman JA, et al. Guidelines for the diagnosis and management of patients with thoracic aortic disease: executive summary. *Circulation* 2010;121:e266-e369.

[47] Vahanian A, Alfieri O, Andreotti F, et al. Joint Task Force on the Management of Valvular Heart Disease of the European Society of Cardiology (ESC); European Association for Cardio-Thoracic Surgery (EACTS). *Eur Heart J.* 2012;33:2451-96.

[48] Etz CD, Misfeld M, Borger MA, Luehr M, Strotdrees E, Mohr FW. Current indications for surgical repair in patients with bicuspid aortic valve and ascending aortic ectasia. *Cardiol Res Pract* 2012.

[49] Park CB, Greason KL, Suri RM, Michelena HI, Schaff HV, Sundt TM. Fate of nonreplaced sinuses of Valsalva in bicuspid aortic valve disease. *J Thorac Cardiovasc Surg* 2011;142:278-84.

[50] Rankin JS, Hammill BG, Ferguson TB, et al. Determinants of operative mortality in valvular heart surgery. *J Thorac Cardiovasc Surg* 2006;131:547-57.

[51] Sundt TM, Mora BN, Moon MR, Bailey MS, Pasque MK, Gay WA. Options for repair of a bicuspid aortic valve and ascending aortic aneurysm. *Ann Thorac Surg* 2000;69:1333-7.

[52] Badiu CC, Bleiziffer S, Eichinger WB, et al. Are bicuspid aortic valves a limitation for aortic valve repair? *Eur J Cardiothorac Surg* 2011;40:1097-104.

[53] Schäfers HJ, Aicher D, Langer F, Lausberg HF. Preservation of the bicuspid aortic valve. *Ann Thorac Surg* 2007;83: S740-5.

In: Bicuspid Aortic Valve
Editor: Anthony Chapman
ISBN: 978-1-63482-786-7

Chapter 2

Genetic Influences on Phenotype in Bicuspid Aortic Valve: Screening, Diagnosis and Prognosis

Catherine Francis and John Pepper
NIHR Cardiovascular BRU, Royal Brompton Hospital; National Heart & Lung Institute, Imperial College London and Institute of Cardiovascular Medicine and Science, London/Liverpool

Abstract

Bicuspid Aortic Valve (BAV) is a condition which displays great phenotypic and genotypic variability; a feature which has hindered identification of discrete genetic influences on phenotype. From a genetic perspective, cases range from those associated with known syndromes, such as Turner or Marfan syndromes, to families in whom classic Mendelian patterns of inheritance are observed, to sporadic *de novo* cases with no clear heritability. In addition, the genetic influences on each individual component of the overall BAV phenotype may be separate and complex. In this chapter, we will review the known syndromes and genetic variants associated with BAV and its complications. We will review genome-wide association studies, linkage analyses and next-generation sequencing studies which are beginning to build a more comprehensive picture of the genetic basis of BAV, and will explore how these genetic variants may interact with haemodynamic factors to create an individual phenotype. We will also review the prospects for developing tools for genetic screening of families and for risk stratification and explore the future steps which are necessary for creation of an individualised approach to managing BAV.

Introduction

The Bicuspid Aortic Valve (BAV) is the most common congenital heart defect, with an estimated prevalence in the general population of 0.5-2% [2, 3]. BAV is known to be heritable, but it displays incomplete penetrance and phenotypic heterogeneity, making genetic studies problematic [1, 4]. The pathophysiology of BAV and of its complications is poorly understood, but it has become increasingly apparent that genetics and haemodynamics interact to produce different manifestations of the disease. Over a third of BAV cases (36.7%) appear to be familial and inherited in Mendelian fashion [5] and yet, even in these apparently "straightforward" cases, the genetic and molecular basis of the disorder has remained elusive. This is not only an academic problem; there is an urgent need for greater knowledge of underlying pathophysiology and risk stratification [1].

Evidence for Heritability of BAV

First degree relatives of patients with BAV have around a 10-fold higher risk of BAV than the general population [5, 6]. The literature reports many multiplex families, in whom BAV follows classical Mendelian inheritance; most commonly autosomal dominant [5]. Classic twin studies to estimate heritability are problematic in the context of congenital heart disease, as the prevalence of all structural cardiac defects is increased around two-fold in monozygotic twins, confounding statistical analysis. Studies have therefore used different methods to estimate heritability.

The prospective screening of families of patients with BAV has determined the prevalence of both BAV itself (around 9-10%) and also other related cardiac abnormalities, such as persistent ductus arteriosus, coarctation of the aorta, ventricular septal defect, thoracic aortic aneurysm or hypoplastic left heart syndrome. One such study by Cripe et al.[7] evaluated 50 probands with BAV and their families; a total of 309 subjects. 32% of the families studied had two or more members with BAV or related congenital cardiovascular disease. The heritability (h^2) of BAV in this cohort was estimated to be 0.89 - ie the vast majority of cases could be explained by genetic transmission alone.

Patterns of inheritance can vary in families, with no single-gene model seeming to explain all the familial cases [1]. This phenotypic and genotypic heterogeneity has greatly increased the difficulties in conducting adequately powered linkage studies, as probands may easily be missed due to subtle forms of phenotypic expression and reduced penetrance. In addition, the majority of BAV cases (over two-thirds), appear to arise as sporadic *"de novo"* forms of disease, with no clear family history identified [4, 5].

The picture becomes even more complicated when one considers the phenotypic heterogeneity of the condition. Multiple genetic alleles seem to interact, causing BAV to co-segregate with other congenital heart defects in some cases [7]. Phenotypes such as hypoplastic left heart syndrome (HLHS) are closely related to BAV, along with abnormalities of the aorta including coarctation and thoracic aortic aneurysm (TAA) [8,9-11]. The latter may even be seen in isolation in families of patients with BAV, even in individuals with a normal tricuspid aortic valve [12, 13]. These related phenotypes represent a broad spectrum of developmental abnormalities of the aorta and outflow tract; whether they represent different manifestations of one entity or multiple separate pathophysiological processes is still uncertain. Of interest is one case report of monochorionic twins who displayed distinct phenotypes [14] - one with HLHS, the other with isolated non-stenotic BAV. It was hypothesised that the genetic substrate must be identical in these twins, and therefore the divergent phenotypes arose solely due to exposure to differing haemodynamic profiles *in utero*. This is certainly a compelling argument and indeed it has long been known that blood flow through the primitive heart during embryonic development plays a crucial role in differentiation of cardiovascular structures. The idea of BAV being a "*forme fruste*" of HLHS is not a new one [10], and there is clear evidence of increased prevalence of HLHS in BAV kindreds. It is likely that multiple influences; some undoubtedly haemodynamic, some genetic and some environmental, interact to determine expressivity in individuals. In the case of the twins, subtle changes in genetics or haemodynamics may have arisen during development, accounting for the phenotypic difference. Whatever the explanation for this particular anomaly, it serves as a good illustration of the subtlety and complexity of the influences on phenotype in BAV, and therefore the difficulty in elucidating the genetic architecture of the condition.

Figure 1 illustrates the different genetic influences on phenotype in BAV. In addition to the "causative" single gene mutations underlying syndromic and inherited forms of BAV, it seems that there are also genetic alleles which act as significant disease modifiers. These may be rare, with large phenotypic effects, such as variants which may cause aortic structural abnormalities; or common polymorphisms, which may, for example, increase susceptibility to aortic "damage" caused by aberrant haemodynamics.

The complexity of BAV genetics means that a variety of different approaches is needed to understand the pathology (see Figure 2). These may be “bottom-up” – examining the molecular pathways involved in normal valve and aortic development to identify likely culprit genes, susceptibility alleles or pathways-or “top-down” – finding families in whom BAV is clearly inherited and using linkage analysis to identify mutations that confer high disease risk. Figure 2 displays the different experimental methods which are needed to elucidate the genetic architecture of BAV, and which underpin the identification of genetic biomarkers and their translation into clinical practice.

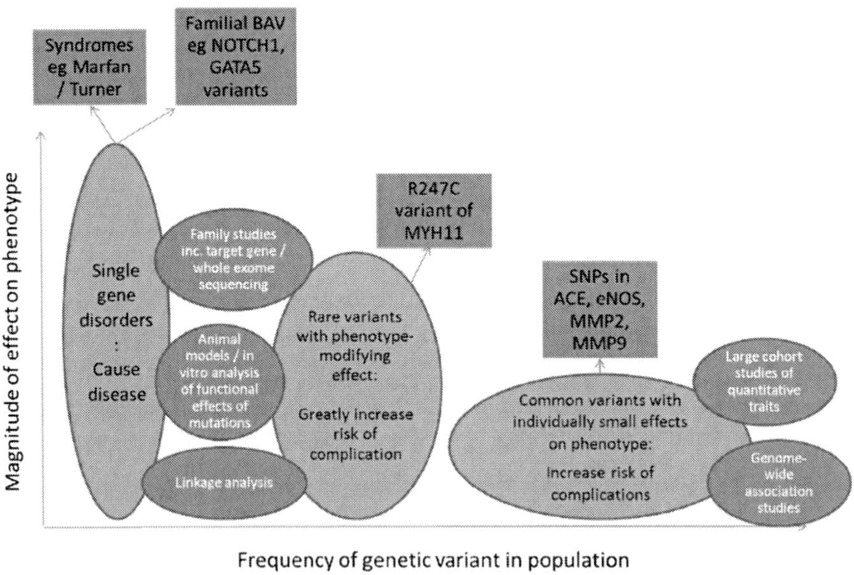

Figure 1. The varied genetic influences on phenotype in BAV, with examples of each, and experimental strategies to identify these variants. Figure based on Prakash et al. 2014 [1].

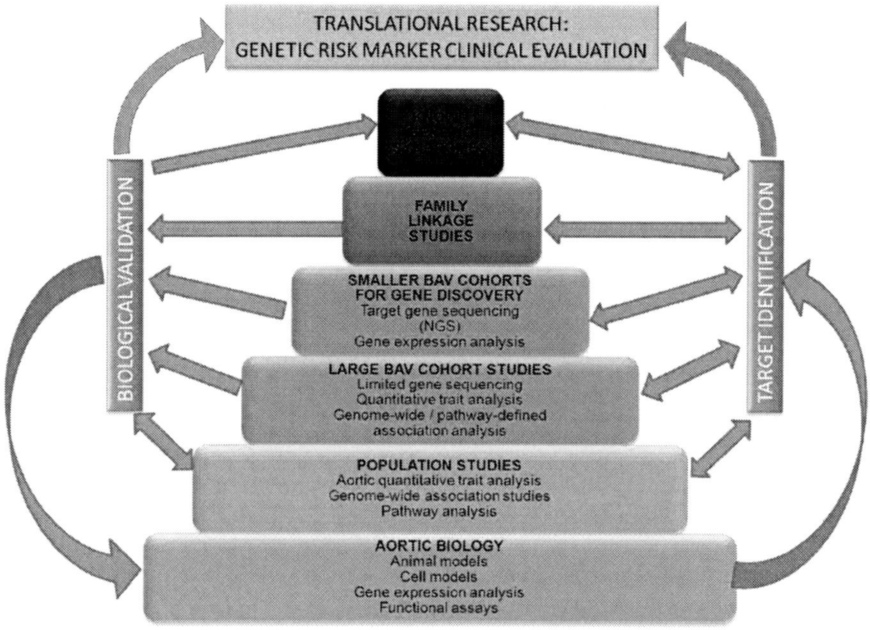

Figure 2. Key to future clinical use of genetic risk markers in BAV is a hierarchy of understanding, founded upon knowledge of aortic biology. Cohort studies and family studies can be informative to identify rare variants, but the linkages established by these methods must be biologically validated to prove causation.

Normal Valve Development

There are multiple different genetic influences on phenotype in BAV. Firstly, there is an underlying developmental abnormality - a defect in the formation or differentiation of the endocardial cushions into the valve leaflets. This underlying abnormality creates a substrate for pathology which may interact with additional genetic or haemodynamic factors to influence eventual phenotype, including thoracic aortic aneurysm or valve dysfunction.

The developmental mechanisms underlying valve formation have been extensively studied. The primitive linear heart tube forms by around 3 weeks in the human embryo, expressing cardiac-specific genes such as *NKX2.5* and *GATA4*. This is followed at weeks 4-5 by looping of the cardiac tube [15]. At around this time, the primary myocardium secretes a gelatinous matrix, called cardiac jelly, forming swellings at the atrioventricular junction and outflow tract [16]. These swellings form the endocardial cushions. The endocardial cells lining the inside surface of the heart tube at these points undergo endothelial-mesenchymal transformation [15]; these cells proliferate and grow inwards, and are joined by both secondary heart field progenitors (positioned in the pharyngeal mesoderm) and migrating cardiac neural crest cells. Contact between the two endocardial cushions results in fusion, followed by formation of the thin valve leaflets. The neural crest cells create a crescent-shaped septal wedge which divides the outflow tract into aortic and pulmonary components [17]. The interaction with neural crest cells and with secondary heart field cells is crucial for normal outflow tract development (see Figure 3). It is hypothesised that defects in the function of each of these contributing cell lineages at different stages of valve and outflow tract development are, in part, responsible for the different phenotypes observed in BAV [18].

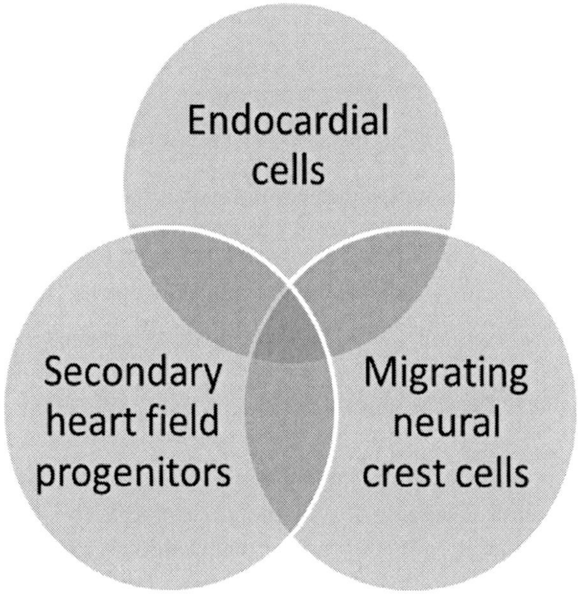

Figure 3. The 3 cell lineages thought to contribute to valvulogenesis & outflow tract development; defects in the function of each may contribute to different phenotypes seen in BAV.

Multiple different signalling pathways are involved in the complex process of valve formation; over a hundred genes have been identified which contribute to the process of endothelial-mesenchymal transformation alone, with most research focussing on chick and mouse embryo development [15,

19-23]. These signalling pathways include those controlled by: Vascular Endothelial Growth Factor (VEGF), Transforming Growth Factor-β (TGF- β), Epidermal Growth Factor (EGF), Notch1, Wnt/B-catenin, Nuclear factor of activated T-cells, cytoplasmic 1 (NFATC1), Mitogen Activated Protein Kinase (MAPK), Fibroblast Growth Factors (FGFs), Bone Morphogenetic Proteins (BMPs), along with transcription factors, including Twist1, Tbx20, Msx1/2, and Sox9 [15, 16, 18, 24, 25]. These are active during early valvulogenesis and maturation of the valve leaflets. The exquisite temporal distribution of these factors, along with cross-talk and interaction between the pathways allows normal valve development. It is no surprise, therefore, that small perturbations in levels of key factors can lead to significant phenotypic aberrations, and these pathways have become the subjects of investigation in BAV.

Animal Models of BAV

An inbred strain of Syrian hamsters demonstrates incomplete penetrance, with fusion of the right and left coronary leaflets of the aortic valve seen in around 58%[26]. These Syrian hamsters display defective outflow tract septation. The cellular origin of the problem is hypothesised to be the neural crest cells which control this process, and which contribute to proximal aortic development. In contrast, *eNOS* knockout mice display fusion of the right- and non-coronary cusps of the aortic valve; a developmental defect which has been shown to be related to the anomalous development of the endocardial cushions themselves. The distinct developmental origins of these differing valve morphologies has been suggested to explain the more severe histopathological changes in aortic walls of patients with right- and left-coronary cusp fusion [18]. Unfortunately, the genetic abnormality in the Syrian hamster strain underlying the BAV phenotype has not been clearly identified.

As we have seen, loss of endothelial nitric oxide synthase function in a mouse model can result in defective valvulogenesis [26]. *eNOS* knockout mice develop a BAV phenotype[27] and, whilst no genetic mutation in *eNOS* has been identified in human BAV, eNOS expression has been found to be lower in the aorta of patients with BAVs [28]. eNOS expression is shear-stress responsive, also creating an interesting theoretical link between the aberrant haemodynamics produced by turbulent flow through a bicuspid valve, and the pathogenetic mechanism itself [16]. One of the *eNOS*-inducing transcription factors, GATA5, has also been implicated in BAV pathogenesis. Evidence for its involvement comes from the *GATA5* knockout mouse, in which there was incomplete penetrance (around 1/4) of a BAV phenotype [29]. GATA5 is expressed in endothelial and endocardial cells, and it is hypothesised that the tight regulation of eNOS levels by GATA5 during endocardial cushion development is vital for normal tricuspid valve formation [30]. Evidence for GATA5 being key in BAV also comes from human studies, in which rare *GATA5* variants in highly-conserved transcriptional activation domains have been associated with BAV [31, 32]. GATA5 works in concert with two other GATA factors: GATA4 and GATA6; defects in which cause varying congenital heart disease in humans. *GATA4/5/6* compound heterozygotes also display severe cardiovascular abnormalities, including BAV.

The *GATA5* knockout mice also have been shown to display reduced NOTCH 1 signalling[29]. Specifically, expression levels of JAG1, the NOTCH ligand, are reduced. *NOTCH1* knockout mice develop severe cardiac malformations, which result in early death, and the pathway is known to be vital for normal cardiac development [23, 33], controlling many different aspects of valvulogenesis. Endothelial-mesenchymal transformation is dependent upon NOTCH1 [23], which also acts as a mediator of signalling between the secondary heart field and migrating neural crest. Therefore, defective NOTCH1 signalling causes BAV and histopathological abnormalities of the aortic wall [34]. NOTCH1 was also the first gene identified as a culprit in families with bicuspid aortic valve, and mutations are associated with increased valve calcification [35]. Mutations in *JAG1*, the gene encoding NOTCH ligand, cause BAV in the context of Alagille syndrome Interestingly, there is significant interaction between the NOTCH1 signalling pathway and both the eNOS pathway (see above) and TGFβ pathway, which is heavily implicated in human aortic disease (see human genetic syndromes, below) [20]. This provides biological plausibility for the involvement of genes in all 3 pathways in development of BAV phenotypes.

Involvement of cells of the cushion mesenchyme in pathogenesis has also been established by the high prevalence of BAV in a mouse model with tissue-specific deletion of *Alk2 (ACVR1)* [36].

Other animal models of BAV formation include the *NKX2-5* haplo-insufficient mouse. *NKX2-5* knockout induces early embryonic lethality, but heterozygous mice display increased prevalence of BAV, at 11%, along with increased incidence of atrial septation defects [37]. There is significant phenotypic heterogeneity in these mice; a finding mirrored in human studies, in which *NKX2-5* has been associated with a broad spectrum of congenital heart disease, from atrial septal defects to severe hypoplastic left heart syndrome [38]. Evidence for the involvement of *NKX2-5* in human disease has been bolstered by the recent identification of a loss-of-function mutation in *NKX2-5* responsible for an autosomal dominant form of BAV [39]. Functional characterisation of this defect again highlights the complex interactions of molecular pathways in pathogenesis, as it inhibited the normal synergism between NKX2-5 and GATA5.

Hoxa1 is a related homeobox gene, which is expressed in the neural crest cells which contribute to aortic valve formation. Homozygous mutations in this gene in humans cause very severe cardiovascular and brainstem abnormalities; and in the mouse, cardiovascular defects include interrupted aortic arch (in 50%), and BAV in 24% [40, 41].

Whilst these animal models have offered some "bottom-up" insight into the molecular and genetic mechanisms which contribute to bicuspid aortic valve formation, they often correlate poorly with genetic abnormalities found in human subjects, where mutations in the genes responsible for BAV in animals account for only a very small number of cases.

Human Genetic Syndromes

Syndromic associations with BAV, such as Marfan and Turner syndromes have provided some clues as to the underlying genetic / molecular basis of the disorder[1, 42]. Some of these syndromes may be incompletely penetrant - or with subtle forms of systemic features, meaning that patients may reach adulthood without a clear diagnosis. The presence of BAV should therefore provide motivation for careful examination for any other systemic features associated with the syndromes summarized in table 1.

30-40% of patients with Turner syndrome have BAV [44], and these patients have a higher than average incidence of associated aortic abnormalities such as aortic coarctation or aneurysm. The link with Turner syndrome, as well as the male preponderance of the condition in the population (at a ratio of around 2:1 male:female) provides some evidence for an X-linked pathogenetic mechanism. However, the genes responsible are unknown.

Table 1. Selected syndromes which may be associated with BAV, adapted and expanded from Canadas et al., 2010 & Prakash et al., 2014 [1, 43]

SYNDROME	PHENOTYPE	GENETIC BASIS
Turner syndrome	TAA, short stature, webbed neck, widely spaced nipples, gonadal dysfunction, BAV, aortic coarctation	45, XO
Marfan syndrome	Aortic root aneurysm, ectopia lentis, skeletal abnormalities, dural ectasia, lung disease	*FBN1*
Loeys-Dietz syndrome	Aneurysm of aortic root and other vessels, aortic tortuosity, hypertelorism, cleft palate or abnormal uvula, craniofacial, skeletal and cutaneous abnormalities, PDA, ASD	*TGFBR1, TGFBR2*
Ehlers-Danlos syndrome Type IV	Spontaneous arterial, intestinal or uterine rupture, characteristic facial appearance, translucent skin with easy bruising, hypermobile joints	*COL3A1*
Arterial tortuosity syndrome	Tortuosity, stenosis, and dilatation of major arteries, joint hypermobility, elongated face, hernias	*SLC2A10*
DiGeorge syndrome	Truncus arteriosus, tetralogy of Fallot, craniofacial defects	*22q11.2* deletion
Alagille syndrome	Characteristic facies, jaundice & skeletal abnormalities	*JAG1*
Familial Thoracic Aortic Aneurysm & Dissection (TAAD)	TAAD, premature coronary artery disease, cerebral aneurysms	*ACTA2*
Andersen-Tawil syndrome	Dysmorphism, cardiac arrhythmias, periodic paralysis	*KCNJ2*
Larsen syndrome	Craniofacial and skeletal defects	*FLNB*
Kabuki syndrome	Mental retardation, hearing loss, coarctation	*KMT2D, KDM6A*

The genes which have been discovered in syndromes associated with BAV can also give us insights into the molecular mechanisms underlying the condition, and therefore identify potential treatment targets. For example, in recent years, TGF-β signalling has been implicated in a range of aortopathies [45-47]. Loeys-Dietz syndrome was found to be caused by specific mutations in genes encoding TGF- β receptors 1 and 2 (*TGFBR1&2*) [45]. In addition, it has been (somewhat controversially) hypothesised that abnormalities in Marfan syndrome may arise not solely due to the physical and structural effects of *fibrillin 1* mutations, but also due to impairment of normal TGF- β sequestration [46, 48, 49]. This failure of sequestration is thought to increase bioavailability of TGF- β, activating its SMAD signalling cascade and increasing expression of matrix metalloproteinases (MMPs), leading to matrix proteolysis [50] and thus further impairment of the elastic properties of the aortic wall. The association of a bicuspid aortic valve with these conditions also implicates TGF-β signalling in the pathogenesis of BAV [51], and indeed reduced expression of fibrillin 1 has been seen in the aorta of patients with BAV [52]. In addition, the mouse model of Marfan syndrome, with targeted deletion of *FBN1*, displays a bicuspid valve phenotype [53]. Levels of MMP 2; a downstream effector of TGF-β signalling, have also been shown to be higher, and levels of TIMP-1 lower in patients with BAV and thoracic aortic aneurysm (TAA) than in patients with a tricuspid valve and TAA [54].

However, the TGF- β signalling pathway certainly does not provide all the answers. No mutation in *TGFBR1* or *TGFBR2* has ever been detected in patients with isolated BAV [55], and even in the context of Marfan syndrome, excitement at identification of a potential new treatment target, using angiotensin II receptor blockers to counteract the increased bioavailability of TGF β, has been considerably diminished by the publication of a trial which showed slightly reduced rates of aortic dilatation, but no changes in any clinical endpoint with losartan treatment [56].

Linkage Analyses

Simplistically, this technique uses marker alleles (common single nucleotide polymorphisms (SNPs)) spaced approximately evenly throughout the genome, and identifies those which segregate most reliably with disease in large multi-generational families. The LOD scores (logarithm of odds) give a very rough idea of the distance between the marker alleles and the unknown disease allele. This technique can therefore describe linkage of particular chromosomal coordinates with disease, but cannot normally identify the specific gene responsible. Usually, examination of the biological role of genes close to a particular marker SNP can identify likely candidates, which can then be examined in more detail through deep sequencing.

Early studies identified a few multiplex families in whom BAV appeared to follow an autosomal pattern of inheritance. Early linkage analysis, focussed on identifying a genetic cause of ventricular arrhythmias, identified a potassium channel gene, *KCNJ2* (Andersen Tawil syndrome) associated with BAV along with other manifestations of the syndrome [57] (see Table 1 above). Subsequently Garg et al. [35] described the first genetic linkage of non-syndromic BAV. In a large multi-generational family, BAV linked with chromosomal region 9q, and further sequencing identified the culprit mutation as a variant in *NOTCH1*. A subsequent multi-family analysis replicated these findings in other families, and also identified three new regions of linkage with BAV; 5q15-21, 13q33-qter and 18q22.1 [58]. In these regions, the genes responsible have not been identified.

Target Gene Approach - Next Generation Sequencing

This approach takes a single gene or panel of genes thought to be associated with disease, and undertakes complete sequencing of those genes. Essentially, genomic DNA is fragmented into multiple short "reads," and amplified by polymerase chain reaction (PCR). The base sequence of these reads is then identified by sequential addition of bases, in a process of massively parallel analysis. Different techniques are available to assess which base has aligned with the reads, including fluorescent labelling. The sequences generated from the reads are then aligned bioinformatically against a reference genome.

Deep sequencing of target genes such as *GATA5* and *NKX2-5* has identified multiple putative pathogenic variants in BAV. *GATA5* sequencing was performed in a cohort of 100 cases of BAV [31]. Four rare, non-synonymous variants were identified, which affect highly conserved transcriptional activation domains, and are therefore likely to be pathological. Subsequent studies have confirmed segregation of *GATA5* mutations with BAV disease [32, 59]. Similar methodology was used to identify the *NKX2-5* mutations described above [39].

There is compelling biological evidence for the importance of both these transcription factors in the pathogenesis of BAV - both from mouse models and also from an understanding of their normal role in cardiac development and valvulogenesis. *In silico* modelling and *in vitro* experiments demonstrate the effects of the identified variants on protein function, and these variants have now been demonstrated segregating with disease in families, completing the picture of their involvement in BAV disease. Next generation sequencing often identifies many variants which may affect amino acid sequence (missense, splice region or radical variants), and therefore this additional step of proving biological significance is crucial for determining pathogenicity.

Examining single patients with disease in great detail has arecently provided further insights into BAV development. Extensive functional analysis of a complex patient with a genetic translocation implicated a mutation affecting Matrin 3 expression in pathogenesis of the cardiovascular phenotype, which included BAV [60]. The potential for mutations in this gene to cause BAV was confirmed in a mouse model. However, the general applicability of this finding in the wider context of BAV has yet to be established.

Genome-Wide Association Studies (GWAS)

This technique uses population-based genotyping, by means of a genome-wide SNP array. The entire genome is "covered" with up to 750,000 SNPs, and the genotype of alleles between these SNPs can be "imputed" by reference to ethnicity-specific reference genomes. Statistical analysis is complex - but essentially, in a similar manner to linkage analysis, identifies "peaks" of statistical significance in the genome which correspond to the phenotype of interest - in this case, bicuspid aortic valve. As the SNPs are spread much more densely through the genome, it is often possible to identify specific genes which may be responsible for phenotype. However, the need for multiple testing correction means that sample sizes required for statistical significance are often huge. To reach statistical power for analysis of a binary trait such as BAV (BAV / unaffected), the numbers of subjects required will be in the tens of thousands.

The phenotypic heterogeneity of BAV and the difficulty in identifying cases (requiring echocardiography and / or long-term follow-up to assess for development of aortic pathology) makes it extremely difficult to conduct such a project in BAV. Also, results will be confounded by the undoubted presence of significant numbers of subjects with unrecognised BAV in the control cohort, and also by the reduced penetrance of the condition. These difficulties mean that this technique has not yet been undertaken. The establishment of large, international consortia such as BAVCon[1] and AortaGen[61] however, make this a real possibility in the near future.

A slightly different approach to classical GWAS was used by Wooten et al.[62] who used network analysis techniques to examine SNPs associated with genes with plausible links with BAV. They identified a haplotype within the *AXIN-1/PDIA2* locus, one within the *Endoglin* gene, and a SNP on chromosome 3 which were all associated with BAV. However, further characterisation of these associations has not been published to date.

Genetic Basis of Thoracic Aortic Aneurysm (TAA) in BAV

TAA is common in patients with BAV, reported in around a half of affected individuals [11]. It is becoming increasingly apparent that both inherent genetic and structural abnormalities of the aortic wall, as well as aberrant haemodynamics, contribute to development of this phenotype. There has been some controversy over the relative importance of these contributing factors and, indeed, the contribution from each may vary from patient to patient [42, 63-65]. As discussed in the section above on normal valve development, there are theories that the common embryological origin of part of the valve structure and ascending aorta from neural crest cells, may explain the aortopathy seen in BAV, with a key role for eNOS identified in the normal maturation of these structures.

The relationship of TAA to BAV remains, however, controversial. Development of TAA may follow the same pattern of inheritance as BAV itself in families [1, 66-68], and in these cases, may represent an inherent part of the "BAV phenotype." But there is emerging evidence that it may instead result from distinct genetic influences. First-degree relatives of patients with BAV have a greatly increased prevalence of TAA over the general population [7, 69]. This increased susceptibility to TAA can occur even in relatives with a normally-functioning, tricuspid aortic valve [13, 70]. Aortic elastic function has also been shown to be diminished in relatives with normal valve phenotype [70]. In addition, quantitative aortic traits including aortic root and ascending aortic diameters have been shown to be heritable, with BAV acting as an independent modifying factor in models of inheritance [71]. These studies are not merely of academic interest; the findings have considerable implications for screening of family members, as even those with a structurally normal valve may require surveillance for development of aortic complications.

In patients with BAV, there is much evidence to suggest an inherent structural abnormality of the aorta. Non-invasive imaging suggests impairment of the elastic properties of the aorta, even before any dilatation becomes apparent [72-78]. Histologically, a pattern of cystic medial necrosis may be seen, analagous to that seen in the aorta of patients with Marfan syndrome. Indeed, reduced expression of fibrillin-1 has been shown in the BAV aorta [52] and, recently, *fibrillin-1* mutations have been seen in patients with BAV without overt Marfanoid features [79].

In addition, factors involved in proteolysis, such as MMP2 and MMP9, along with their tissue inhibitors, display distinct expression patterns in the aortas of BAV patients, even in the absence of significant aortic dilatation [54, 80-83]. One transcriptomic study found that the differential gene expression in dilated vs non-dilated aortas in patients with bicuspid valve was different to that seen in patients with tricuspid valve [84]. This suggests a different mechanism of aortic dilatation in BAV.

Candidate genes for TAA development in the context of BAV include *FBN1*, as described above. Another candidate is *MYH11*, which encodes myosin heavy chain, one of the key proteins in the vascular smooth muscle cell contractile apparatus. This has been linked to familial TAA associated with persistent ductus arteriosus and, less frequently, BAV [85, 86]. *MYH11* mutations such as R247C seem also to act as phenotype modifiers, representing a susceptibility trait where this particular variant increases risk of aortic abnormalities, but is not sufficient, in itself, to cause major aortic complications [87, 88].

Thoracic Aortic Aneurysm Associated with BAV: Haemodynamic Theory

The differing susceptibility of the aorta to dilatation in patients with different BAV morphologies has been one argument in favour of a haemodynamic basis for TAA [65, 89]. It is increasingly recognised that different BAV morphologies expose the aortic wall to differing patterns of shear stress and stretch [90-93], and that this, in addition to inherent genetic abnormalities, accounts for aortic wall "weakening" and aneurysm development.

In vitro, human endothelial cells demonstrate different patterns of gene expression in response to differing shear stress [94-96]; a response which alters the underlying properties of the endothelium and the vascular smooth muscle. These both regulate the structure and elastic function of the aortic wall through synthetic, secretory, contractile and structural capabilities. It is increasingly recognised that, even in the absence of classically defined "valve dysfunction," flow patterns in the aortic root and ascending aorta are abnormal in patients with BAV [97]. Furthermore, these flow patterns are distinct between morphological subtypes of BAV [90], providing a mechanistic explanation for the different natural history seen in these subtypes. R-L coronary cusp fusion is associated with dilatation of the aortic root at a younger age and R-N cusp fusion is associated with increased aortic arch dimensions.

It is also proposed that haemodynamics play a crucial role in embryonic development, with flow patterns through the primitive valve structures altering phenotypic expression [98-101]. This is borne out by experiments in our group demonstrating differential expression of genes involved in cardiovascular development in endothelial cells subjected to different patterns of shear stress (Francis et al., submitted for publication). Also, in the case of twins described above [14], it seems that altered haemodynamic conditions in utero may be the explanation for the divergent phenotypes seen.

The relevance of shear stress to aortic disease comes from several directions. Firstly, haemodynamic influences are thought to be of vital importance in cardiovascular system development. Indeed, it has been shown that shear-responsive genes *KLF2*, *eNOS* and *ET-1* play a key role in the development of the cardiovascular system [98]. Therefore, it is conceivable that pathological changes in the genes responsible for shear stress response could cause structural aortic abnormalities. Secondly, the aortopathy seen in BAV is known to represent a complex interplay between haemodynamic and genetic factors [11]; an interplay which is likely to be mediated by the vascular endothelial cells which are the primary mechanosensors of shear stress [11, 102, 103] Thirdly, evidence shows changes in gene expression in the BAV aorta of several genes known to be regulated by flow, such as *eNOS* [104], *MMP*s [82, 105, 106], *PKD-2* [107] and genes in the TGF-β signalling pathway. *eNOS* knockout mice have a high incidence of bicuspid aortic valve [27]. Also, endothelial function has been shown to be impaired in patients with BAV [108]. These pieces of evidence together indicate that endothelial response to altered patterns of shear stress in BAV may be at least in part responsible for the aortopathy seen in that condition. Therefore, understanding the normal endothelial response to shear is vital for understanding how this process may malfunction in the diseased aorta.

Studies of haemodynamic abnormalities in BAV certainly provide compelling evidence for the involvement of flow-regulated mechanisms in disease; the "controversy" in the literature over haemodynamics versus genetics seems a rather false one; it is evident that both contribute to phenotype, and interact in complex and profound ways, both during development and throughout adult life. The real questions lie in unraveling the mechanisms underlying the aortic response to the particular haemodynamic challenges of BAV.

Genotype-Phenotype Correlations

We know that individual genotypes confer different risks of complications in BAV. Figure 1 is a schematic representation of the different types of genetic influence on phenotype. The most profound examples of specific genotype-phenotype correlations are the variants associated with known syndromes. For example, in Turner syndrome, loss of the second X chromosome appears to confer a greatly increased risk of aortic complications in patients with BAV, with increased rates of thoracic aortic aneurysm and dissection[44, 109, 110]. The practical implications of this are clear - these patients will require meticulous follow-up and a lower threshold for intervention on the ascending aorta and aortic root is appropriate.

Other phenotypic modifiers may have profound effects - such as the R247C variant in *MYH11*, which is known to modify aortic biomechanical properties [87, 88], but which is likely to require a further insult - be it genetic, "environmental" or haemodynamic - to engender significant aortopathy.

More recently, *NOTCH1* mutations have been hypothesised to produce a phenotype distinct from other forms of familial BAV. In patients with *NOTCH1* mutations, the predominant clinical feature is of calcific and dysfunctional aortic valve, with low incidence of coexisting TAA. In the original paper by Garg et al. [35], a clear link was identified between inactivating mutations in *NOTCH1* and autosomal dominant valve disease. 4 out of 9 affected individuals had TAA. However, there was one individual who had TAA without valve disease - ie he had a normally-functioning, tricuspid aortic valve, and did not have the familial *NOTCH1* mutation. This finding, strengthened by subsequent genotype-phenotype correlations in BAV, implies two distinct mechanisms of expressivity - one (*NOTCH1*) for calcific valve disease, and the other for highly penetrant TAA with uncommon valve calcification [35, 111].

Phenotype Modifiers - Common Variants

Other modifiers may have much more subtle effects on phenotype - and are common variants in the rest of the population. Identification of these variants is problematic, and requires large-scale GWAS analysis of quantitative traits such as aortic dimensions, to identify variants which could also act in the context of aortic disease to affect complications. A target gene approach has, however, identified several common polymorphisms which may have small individual effects on phenotype but which, taken together, may explain some of the inter-individual differences seen in expression. SNPs in *eNOS* and *ACE* (angiotensin converting enzyme) have been shown to influence aortic aneurysm risk in BAV patients, as have SNPs in *MMP2* and *MMP9* [105, 112-114].

microRNAs: The New Kids on the Block

MicroRNAs are short, single-stranded RNA molecules, approximately 22 nucleotides in length, which are responsible for post-transcriptional inhibition of gene expression. They prevent the translation of other messenger RNA molecules, by binding to sequences at the 3' untranslated region (UTR) of messenger RNA molecules.

miRNA29 is known to regulate elastin and other extracellular matrix proteins during cardiac and aortic development [115, 116]. Boon et al. [116] demonstrated an increase in its expression following angiotensin II infusion in mice (a model of aortic aneurysm formation), and a corresponding decrease in expression of elastin and other ECM components. They also found increased expression in aortas of mouse models of genetic aortopathy. Treatment with an inhibitor of miRNA29 was able to abrogate the angiotensin-II induced increase in aortic diameter. Significantly, they were also able to demonstrate an increased level of miRNA29 in human aneurysmal aortic tissue from patients with both BAV and with normal tricuspid valve (TAV). miRNA1 and miRNA21 have also been found to be differentially expressed in BAV versus TAV aortas [80].

Given the clear regulatory effects of miRNA on aortic biology, and the evidence for differential expression in BAV versus TAV, it seems likely that miRNAs contribute to phenotype in this condition, although there is no proof as yet, and we have a very primitive understanding of the mechanisms of control of microRNA expression.

State of Knowledge

Despite advances in our understanding of the biological pathways involved in valvulogenesis, identification of genetic variants causative of syndromes associated with BAV, and identification of genes in which mutations can cause sporadic BAV, there remains a huge amount of "missing" heritability.

We studied 177 unrelated patients with BAV without known syndromic basis, recruited from 2 tertiary centres (Francis et al., submitted to Heart Valve Society Conference 2015), and were able to identify a causative genetic variant in just 9% of our cohort. *In silico* modelling identified likely pathological variants in candidate genes in a further 31% of patients with known family history - but this modelling is far from proof of pathological causation. This leaves the vast majority of cases of BAV unexplained, even in those families where there is a clear genetic link.

Work from large genetic consortia aims to clarify the role of genetics in BAV, using all of the methods described above, with the aim of building a comprehensive picture of the genetic architecture of the condition.

Conclusion

Genetic screening for BAV has clear potential benefits, with the goal of "stratified medicine," whereby an individual's treatment may be tailored to his or her genetic and clinical profile. However, the state of our knowledge is not yet sufficiently advanced to develop a "one-size-fits-all" screening and risk evaluation strategy. It has only been recently that guidelines have recommended screening of family members at all [12, 117]. Medics in general are often poor at communicating uncertainty in counselling patients about risks, and there is a general reluctance in cardiac and cardiothoracic surgical clinics to broach subjects of family screening, reproductive risk and long-term prognosis. New services which create a clinical framework for family screening with a comprehensive imaging and genetic assessment are being established, but the interpretation of test results is not a trivial task, and specialist genetic assessment and counselling is required [1, 66].

The uncertainties of risk assessment are great, and screening often raises more questions than it answers. Is a patient's brother with a structurally normal valve and aorta free from disease? Should the brother be screened at regular intervals throughout his life? How would identification of a likely causative genetic variant change this advice? These are all questions with no correct answers; the appropriate response is likely to entail a detailed discussion with the patient and family about the risks and uncertainties involved. In an adult first-degree relative with a structurally completely normal (tricuspid) valve and normal aortic dimensions, the risk of developing severe complications later in life is likely to be minimal - but not zero. Genetic screening may have some bearing on this risk assessment. If mutations are identified in the family which segregate with disease, are low-risk for thoracic aortic aneurysm (eg *NOTCH1*), and are not found in the relative in question, then it is likely appropriate to discharge the relative from follow-up. However, if there is any question about the genotype-phenotype correlation in that particular family, if variants are identified in "high risk" genes for aortic complications, such as *MYH11*, *ACTA2*, *FBN1*, *TGFBR1* or *TGFBR2*, of if there is highly penetrant aortic disease in other family members, then long-term follow-up would be appropriate.

Even one-time screening of family members has significant resource implications for healthcare systems; the suggestion of a requirement for repeated screening is even more daunting. However, it is hoped that future genetic studies will elucidate further the genetic architecture of the condition, allowing more effective risk stratification. No single experimental model will allow this; the integration of findings from major international clinical research consortia, individual case reports and basic science experiments will all be key. It is often said that one should not end a discourse by stating that further research is needed, but given the very primitive state of our understanding of the genetic basis of BAV it is hard to see how else to conclude.

References

[1] Prakash, SK; Bosse, Y; Muehlschlegel, JD; Michelena, HI; Limongelli, G; Della, Corte, A; et al. A roadmap to investigate the genetic basis of bicuspid aortic valve and its complications: insights from the International BAVCon (Bicuspid Aortic Valve Consortium). *Journal of the American College of Cardiology*. 2014, 64(8), 832-9.

[2] Basso, C; Boschello, M; Perrone, C; Mecenero, A; Cera, A; Bicego, D; et al. An echocardiographic survey of primary school children for bicuspid aortic valve. *The American journal of cardiology*. 2004, 93(5), 661-3.

[3] Braverman, AC; Guven, H; Beardslee, MA; Makan, M; Kates, AM; Moon, MR. The bicuspid aortic valve. *Current problems in cardiology*. 2005, 30(9), 470-522.

[4] Siu, SC; Silversides, CK. Bicuspid aortic valve disease. *Journal of the American College of Cardiology*. 2010, 55(25), 2789-800.

[5] Huntington, K; Hunter, AG; Chan, KL. A prospective study to assess the frequency of familial clustering of congenital bicuspid aortic valve. *Journal of the American College of Cardiology*. 1997, 30(7), 1809-12.

[6] Panayotova, R; Macnab, A; Waterworth, PD. A pilot project of familial screening in patients with bicuspid aortic valve disease. *The Journal of heart valve disease*. 2013, 22(2), 150-5.

[7] Cripe, L; Andelfinger, G; Martin, LJ; Shooner, K; Benson, DW. Bicuspid aortic valve is heritable. *Journal of the American College of Cardiology*. 2004, 44(1), 138-43.

[8] Duran, AC; Frescura, C; Sans-Coma, V; Angelini, A; Basso, C; Thiene, G. Bicuspid aortic valves in hearts with other congenital heart disease. *The Journal of heart valve disease*. 1995, 4(6), 581-90.

[9] Hinton, RB; Martin, LJ; Rame-Gowda, S; Tabangin, ME; Cripe, LH; Benson, DW. Hypoplastic left heart syndrome links to chromosomes 10q and 6q and is genetically related to bicuspid aortic valve. *Journal of the American College of Cardiology*. 2009, 53(12), 1065-71.

[10] McBride, KL; Pignatelli, R; Lewin, M; Ho, T; Fernbach, S; Menesses, A; et al. Inheritance analysis of congenital left ventricular outflow tract obstruction malformations: Segregation, multiplex relative risk, and heritability. *American journal of medical genetics Part A*. 2005, 134A(2), 180-6.

[11] Tadros, TM; Klein, MD; Shapira, OM. Ascending aortic dilatation associated with bicuspid aortic valve: pathophysiology, molecular biology, and clinical implications. *Circulation*. 2009, 119(6), 880-90.

[12] Hiratzka, LF; Bakris, GL; Beckman, JA; Bersin, RM; Carr, VF; Casey, DE; Jr; et al. 2010 ACCF/AHA/AATS/ACR/ASA/SCA/SCAI/SIR/STS/SVM Guidelines for the diagnosis and management of patients with thoracic aortic disease. A Report of the American College of Cardiology Foundation/American Heart Association Task Force on Practice Guidelines, American Association for Thoracic Surgery, American College of Radiology,American Stroke Association, Society of Cardiovascular Anesthesiologists, Society for Cardiovascular Angiography and Interventions, Society of Interventional Radiology, Society of Thoracic Surgeons,and Society for Vascular Medicine. *Journal of the American College of Cardiology*. 2010, 55(14), e27-e129.

[13] Loscalzo, ML; Goh, DL; Loeys, B; Kent, KC; Spevak, PJ; Dietz, HC. Familial thoracic aortic dilation and bicommissural aortic valve: a prospective analysis of natural history and inheritance. *American journal of medical genetics Part A*. 2007, 143A(17), 1960-7.

[14] Mu, TS; McAdams, RM; Bush, DM. A case of hypoplastic left heart syndrome and bicuspid aortic valve in monochorionic twins. *Pediatric cardiology*. 2005, 26(6), 884-5.

[15] Gittenberger-de, Groot, AC; Bartelings, MM; Deruiter, MC; Poelmann, RE. Basics of cardiac development for the understanding of congenital heart malformations. *Pediatric research*. 2005, 57(2), 169-76.

[16] Laforest, B; Nemer, M. Genetic insights into bicuspid aortic valve formation. *Cardiology research and practice*. 2012, 2012:180297.

[17] Phillips, HM; Mahendran, P; Singh, E; Anderson, RH; Chaudhry, B; Henderson, DJ. Neural crest cells are required for correct positioning of the developing outflow cushions and pattern the arterial valve leaflets. *Cardiovascular research*. 2013, 99(3), 452-60.

[18] Grewal, N; DeRuiter, MC; Jongbloed, MR; Goumans, MJ; Klautz, RJ; Poelmann, RE; et al. Normal and abnormal development of the aortic wall and valve: correlation with clinical entities. *Netherlands heart journal: monthly journal of the Netherlands Society of Cardiology and the Netherlands Heart Foundation*. 2014, 22(9), 363-9.

[19] Chang, AC; Fu, Y; Garside, VC; Niessen, K; Chang, L; Fuller, M; et al. Notch initiates the endothelial-to-mesenchymal transition in the atrioventricular canal through autocrine activation of soluble guanylyl cyclase. *Developmental cell*. 2011, 21(2), 288-300.

[20] Fu, Y; Chang, A; Chang, L; Niessen, K; Eapen, S; Setiadi, A; et al. Differential regulation of transforming growth factor beta signaling pathways by Notch in human endothelial cells. *The Journal of biological chemistry*. 2009, 284(29), 19452-62.

[21] Niessen, K; Karsan, A. Notch signaling in the developing cardiovascular system. *American journal of physiology Cell physiology*. 2007, 293(1), C1-11.

[22] Noseda, M; McLean, G; Niessen, K; Chang, L; Pollet, I; Montpetit, R; et al. Notch activation results in phenotypic and functional changes consistent with endothelial-to-mesenchymal transformation. *Circulation research*. 2004, 94(7), 910-7.

[23] Timmerman, LA; Grego-Bessa, J; Raya, A; Bertran, E; Perez-Pomares, JM; Diez, J; et al. Notch promotes epithelial-mesenchymal transition during cardiac development and oncogenic transformation. *Genes & development*. 2004, 18(1), 99-115.

[24] Chakraborty, S; Combs, MD; Yutzey, KE. Transcriptional regulation of heart valve progenitor cells. *Pediatric cardiology*. 2010, 31(3), 414-21.

[25] Combs, MD; Yutzey, KE. Heart valve development: regulatory networks in development and disease. *Circulation research*. 2009, 105(5), 408-21.

[26] Sans-Coma, V; Carmen, Fernandez, M; Fernandez, B; Duran, AC; Anderson, RH; Arque, JM. Genetically alike Syrian hamsters display both bifoliate and trifoliate aortic valves. *Journal of anatomy*. 2012, 220(1), 92-101.

[27] Lee, TC; Zhao, YD; Courtman, DW; Stewart, DJ. Abnormal aortic valve development in mice lacking endothelial nitric oxide synthase. *Circulation*. 2000, 101(20), 2345-8.

[28] Aicher, D; Urbich, C; Zeiher, A; Dimmeler, S; Schafers, HJ. Endothelial nitric oxide synthase in bicuspid aortic valve disease. *The Annals of thoracic surgery*. 2007, 83(4), 1290-4.

[29] Laforest, B; Andelfinger, G; Nemer, M. Loss of Gata5 in mice leads to bicuspid aortic valve. *The Journal of clinical investigation*. 2011, 121(7), 2876-87.

[30] Nemer, G; Nemer, M. Cooperative interaction between GATA5 and NF-ATc regulates endothelial-endocardial differentiation of cardiogenic cells. *Development*. 2002, 129(17), 4045-55.

[31] Padang, R; Bagnall, RD; Richmond, DR; Bannon, PG; Semsarian, C. Rare non-synonymous variations in the transcriptional activation

domains of GATA5 in bicuspid aortic valve disease. *Journal of molecular and cellular cardiology*. 2012, 53(2), 277-81.

[32] Foffa, I; Ait, Ali, L; Panesi, P; Mariani, M; Festa, P; Botto, N; et al. Sequencing of NOTCH1, GATA5, TGFBR1 and TGFBR2 genes in familial cases of bicuspid aortic valve. *BMC medical genetics*. 2013, 14:44.

[33] Niessen, K; Karsan, A. Notch signaling in cardiac development. *Circulation research*. 2008, 102(10), 1169-81.

[34] Jain, D; Dietz, HC; Oswald, GL; Maleszewski, JJ; Halushka, MK. Causes and histopathology of ascending aortic disease in children and young adults. *Cardiovascular pathology: the official journal of the Society for Cardiovascular Pathology*. 2011, 20(1), 15-25.

[35] Garg, V; Muth, AN; Ransom, JF; Schluterman, MK; Barnes, R; King, IN; et al. Mutations in NOTCH1 cause aortic valve disease. *Nature*. 2005, 437(7056), 270-4.

[36] Thomas, PS; Sridurongrit, S; Ruiz-Lozano, P; Kaartinen, V. Deficient signaling via Alk2 (Acvr1) leads to bicuspid aortic valve development. *PloS one*. 2012, 7(4), e35539.

[37] Biben, C; Weber, R; Kesteven, S; Stanley, E; McDonald, L; Elliott, DA; et al. Cardiac septal and valvular dysmorphogenesis in mice heterozygous for mutations in the homeobox gene Nkx2-5. *Circulation research*. 2000, 87(10), 888-95.

[38] Elliott, DA; Kirk, EP; Yeoh, T; Chandar, S; McKenzie, F; Taylor, P; et al. Cardiac homeobox gene NKX2-5 mutations and congenital heart disease: associations with atrial septal defect and hypoplastic left heart syndrome. *Journal of the American College of Cardiology*. 2003, 41(11), 2072-6.

[39] Qu, XK; Qiu, XB; Yuan, F; Wang, J; Zhao, CM; Liu, XY; et al. A novel NKX2.5 loss-of-function mutation associated with congenital bicuspid aortic valve. *The American journal of cardiology*. 2014, 114(12), 1891-5.

[40] Makki, N; Capecchi, MR. Cardiovascular defects in a mouse model of HOXA1 syndrome. *Human molecular genetics*. 2012, 21(1), 26-31.

[41] Makki, N; Capecchi, MR. Hoxa1 lineage tracing indicates a direct role for Hoxa1 in the development of the inner ear, the heart, and the third rhombomere. *Developmental biology*. 2010, 341(2), 499-509.

[42] Abdulkareem, N; Smelt, J; Jahangiri, M. Bicuspid aortic valve aortopathy: genetics, pathophysiology and medical therapy. *Interactive cardiovascular and thoracic surgery*. 2013, 17(3), 554-9.

[43] Canadas, V; Vilacosta, I; Bruna, I; Fuster, V. Marfan syndrome. Part 1: pathophysiology and diagnosis. *Nature reviews Cardiology*. 2010, 7(5), 256-65.

[44] Kim, HK; Gottliebson, W; Hor, K; Backeljauw, P; Gutmark-Little, I; Salisbury, SR; et al. Cardiovascular anomalies in Turner syndrome: spectrum, prevalence, and cardiac MRI findings in a pediatric and young adult population. *AJR American journal of roentgenology*. 2011, 196(2), 454-60.

[45] Loeys, BL; Chen, J; Neptune, ER; Judge, DP; Podowski, M; Holm, T; et al. A syndrome of altered cardiovascular, craniofacial, neurocognitive and skeletal development caused by mutations in TGFBR1 or TGFBR2. *Nature genetics*. 2005, 37(3), 275-81.

[46] Matt, P; Schoenhoff, F; Habashi, J; Holm, T; Van, Erp, C; Loch, D; et al. Circulating transforming growth factor-beta in Marfan syndrome. *Circulation*. 2009, 120(6), 526-32.

[47] Renard, M; Callewaert, B; Baetens, M; Campens, L; MacDermot, K; Fryns, JP; et al. Novel MYH11 and ACTA2 mutations reveal a role for enhanced TGFbeta signaling in FTAAD. *International journal of cardiology*. 2013, 165(2), 314-21.

[48] Bolar, N; Van, Laer, L; Loeys, BL. Marfan syndrome: from gene to therapy. *Current opinion in pediatrics*. 2012, 24(4), 498-504.

[49] Loeys, BL; Mortier, G; Dietz, HC. Bone lessons from Marfan syndrome and related disorders: fibrillin, TGF-B and BMP at the balance of too long and too short. *Pediatric endocrinology reviews: PER*. 2013, 10 Suppl 2:417-23.

[50] Carta, L; Smaldone, S; Zilberberg, L; Loch, D; Dietz, HC; Rifkin, DB; et al. p38 MAPK is an early determinant of promiscuous Smad2/3 signaling in the aortas of fibrillin-1 (Fbn1)-null mice. *The Journal of biological chemistry*. 2009, 284(9), 5630-6.

[51] Gomez, D; Al, Haj, Zen, A; Borges, LF; Philippe, M; Gutierrez, PS; Jondeau, G; et al. Syndromic and non-syndromic aneurysms of the human ascending aorta share activation of the Smad2 pathway. *The Journal of pathology*. 2009, 218(1), 131-42.

[52] Fedak, PW; de Sa, MP; Verma, S; Nili, N; Kazemian, P; Butany, J; et al. Vascular matrix remodeling in patients with bicuspid aortic valve malformations: implications for aortic dilatation. *The Journal of thoracic and cardiovascular surgery*. 2003, 126(3), 797-806.

[53] Pereira, L; Andrikopoulos, K; Tian, J; Lee, SY; Keene, DR; Ono, R; et al. Targetting of the gene encoding fibrillin-1 recapitulates the vascular aspect of Marfan syndrome. *Nature genetics*. 1997, 17(2), 218-22.

[54] Rabkin, SW. Differential expression of MMP-2, MMP-9 and TIMP proteins in thoracic aortic aneurysm - comparison with and without bicuspid aortic valve: a meta-analysis. *VASA Zeitschrift fur Gefasskrankheiten*. 2014, 43(6), 433-42.

[55] Arrington, CB; Sower, CT; Chuckwuk, N; Stevens, J; Leppert, MF; Yetman, AT; et al. Absence of TGFBR1 and TGFBR2 mutations in patients with bicuspid aortic valve and aortic dilation. *The American journal of cardiology*. 2008, 102(5), 629-31.

[56] Groenink, M; den, Hartog, AW; Franken, R; Radonic, T; de, Waard, V; Timmermans, J; et al. Losartan reduces aortic dilatation rate in adults with Marfan syndrome: a randomized controlled trial. *European heart journal*. 2013, 34(45), 3491-500.

[57] Andelfinger, G; Tapper, AR; Welch, RC; Vanoye, CG; George, AL; Jr. Benson, DW. KCNJ2 mutation results in Andersen syndrome with sex-specific cardiac and skeletal muscle phenotypes. *American journal of human genetics*. 2002, 71(3), 663-8.

[58] Martin, LJ; Ramachandran, V; Cripe, LH; Hinton, RB; Andelfinger, G; Tabangin, M; et al. Evidence in favor of linkage to human chromosomal regions 18q, 5q and 13q for bicuspid aortic valve and associated cardiovascular malformations. *Human genetics*. 2007, 121(2), 275-84.

[59] Bonachea, EM; Chang, SW; Zender, G; LaHaye, S; Fitzgerald-Butt, S; McBride, KL; et al. Rare GATA5 sequence variants identified in individuals with bicuspid aortic valve. *Pediatric research*. 2014, 76(2), 211-6.

[60] Quintero-Rivera, F; Xi, QJ; Keppler-Noreuil, KM; Lee, JH; Higgins, AW; Anchan, RM; et al. MATR3 Disruption in Human and Mouse Associated with Bicuspid Aortic Valve, Aortic Coarctation and Patent Ductus Arteriosus. *Human molecular genetics*. 2015.

[61] Mitchell, GF; Verwoert, GC; Tarasov, KV; Isaacs, A; Smith, AV; Yasmin; et al. Common genetic variation in the 3'-BCL11B gene desert is associated with carotid-femoral pulse wave velocity and excess cardiovascular disease risk: the AortaGen Consortium. *Circulation Cardiovascular genetics*. 2012, 5(1), 81-90.

[62] Wooten, EC; Iyer, LK; Montefusco, MC; Hedgepeth, AK; Payne, DD; Kapur, NK; et al. Application of gene network analysis techniques

identifies AXIN1/PDIA2 and endoglin haplotypes associated with bicuspid aortic valve. *PloS one*. 2010, 5(1), e8830.

[63] Charitos, EI; Stierle, U; Petersen, M; Mohamed, SA; Hanke, T; Schmidtke, C; et al. The fate of the bicuspid valve aortopathy after aortic valve replacement. *European journal of cardio-thoracic surgery: official journal of the European Association for Cardio-thoracic Surgery*. 2014, 45(5), e128-35.

[64] Forte, A; Della, Corte, A; Grossi, M; Bancone, C; Provenzano, R; Finicelli, M; et al. Early cell changes and TGFbeta pathway alterations in the aortopathy associated with bicuspid aortic valve stenosis. *Clinical science*. 2013, 124(2), 97-108.

[65] Kim, YG; Sun, BJ; Park, GM; Han, S; Kim, DH; Song, JM; et al. Aortopathy and bicuspid aortic valve: haemodynamic burden is main contributor to aortic dilatation. *Heart*. 2012, 98(24), 1822-7.

[66] Michelena, HI; Prakash, SK; Della, Corte, A; Bissell, MM; Anavekar, N; Mathieu, P; et al. Bicuspid aortic valve: identifying knowledge gaps and rising to the challenge from the International Bicuspid Aortic Valve Consortium (BAVCon). *Circulation*. 2014, 129(25), 2691-704.

[67] Milewicz, DM; Regalado, ES; Shendure, J; Nickerson, DA; Guo, DC. Successes and challenges of using whole exome sequencing to identify novel genes underlying an inherited predisposition for thoracic aortic aneurysms and acute aortic dissections. *Trends in cardiovascular medicine*. 2014, 24(2), 53-60.

[68] Robinson, PN; Arteaga-Solis, E; Baldock, C; Collod-Beroud, G; Booms, P; De, Paepe, A; et al. The molecular genetics of Marfan syndrome and related disorders. *Journal of medical genetics*. 2006, 43(10), 769-87.

[69] Hinton, RB; Jr., Martin LJ, Tabangin ME, Mazwi ML, Cripe LH, Benson DW. Hypoplastic left heart syndrome is heritable. *Journal of the American College of Cardiology*. 2007, 50(16), 1590-5.

[70] Biner, S; Rafique, AM; Ray, I; Cuk, O; Siegel, RJ; Tolstrup, K. Aortopathy is prevalent in relatives of bicuspid aortic valve patients. *Journal of the American College of Cardiology*. 2009, 53(24), 2288-95.

[71] Martin, LJ; Hinton, RB; Zhang, X; Cripe, LH; Benson, DW. Aorta Measurements are Heritable and Influenced by Bicuspid Aortic Valve. *Frontiers in genetics*. 2011, 2, 61.

[72] Bilen, E; Akcay, M; Bayram, NA; Kocak, U; Kurt, M; Tanboga, IH; et al. Aortic elastic properties and left ventricular diastolic function in patients with isolated bicuspid aortic valve. *The Journal of heart valve disease*. 2012, 21(2), 189-94.

[73] de Wit, A; Vis, K; Jeremy, RW. Aortic stiffness in heritable aortopathies: relationship to aneurysm growth rate. *Heart, lung & circulation*. 2013, 22(1), 3-11.
[74] Gurses, D; Ozyurek, AR; Levent, E; Ulger, Z. Elastic properties of the abdominal aorta in the children with bicuspid aortic valve: an observational study. *Anadolu kardiyoloji dergisi: AKD = the Anatolian journal of cardiology*. 2012, 12(5), 413-9.
[75] Nistri, S; Sorbo, MD; Basso, C; Thiene, G. Bicuspid aortic valve: abnormal aortic elastic properties. *The Journal of heart valve disease*. 2002, 11(3), 369-73, discussion 73-4.
[76] Oulego-Erroz, I; Alonso-Quintela, P; Mora-Matilla, M; Gautreaux, Minaya, S; Lapena-Lopez, de, Armentia, S. Ascending aorta elasticity in children with isolated bicuspid aortic valve. *International journal of cardiology*. 2013, 168(2), 1143-6.
[77] Pees, C; Michel-Behnke, I. Morphology of the bicuspid aortic valve and elasticity of the adjacent aorta in children. *The American journal of cardiology*. 2012, 110(9), 1354-60.
[78] Pichamuthu, JE; Phillippi, JA; Cleary, DA; Chew, DW; Hempel, J; Vorp, DA; et al. Differential tensile strength and collagen composition in ascending aortic aneurysms by aortic valve phenotype. *The Annals of thoracic surgery*. 2013, 96(6), 2147-54.
[79] Pepe, G; Nistri, S; Giusti, B; Sticchi, E; Attanasio, M; Porciani, C; et al. Identification of fibrillin 1 gene mutations in patients with bicuspid aortic valve (BAV) without Marfan syndrome. *BMC medical genetics*. 2014, 15, 23.
[80] Ikonomidis, JS; Ivey, CR; Wheeler, JB; Akerman, AW; Rice, A; Patel, RK; et al. Plasma biomarkers for distinguishing etiologic subtypes of thoracic aortic aneurysm disease. *The Journal of thoracic and cardiovascular surgery*. 2013, 145(5), 1326-33.
[81] Ikonomidis, JS; Ruddy, JM; Benton, SM; Jr., Arroyo J, Brinsa TA, Stroud RE, et al. Aortic dilatation with bicuspid aortic valves: cusp fusion correlates to matrix metalloproteinases and inhibitors. *The Annals of thoracic surgery*. 2012, 93(2), 457-63.
[82] LeMaire, SA; Wang, X; Wilks, JA; Carter, SA; Wen, S; Won, T; et al. Matrix metalloproteinases in ascending aortic aneurysms: bicuspid versus trileaflet aortic valves. *The Journal of surgical research*. 2005, 123(1), 40-8.
[83] Mohamed, SA; Noack, F; Schoellermann, K; Karluss, A; Radtke, A; Schult-Badusche, D; et al. Elevation of matrix metalloproteinases in

different areas of ascending aortic aneurysms in patients with bicuspid and tricuspid aortic valves. *TheScientificWorldJournal*. 2012, 2012: 806261.

[84] Folkersen, L; Wagsater, D; Paloschi, V; Jackson, V; Petrini, J; Kurtovic, S; et al. Unraveling divergent gene expression profiles in bicuspid and tricuspid aortic valve patients with thoracic aortic dilatation: the ASAP study. *Molecular medicine*. 2011, 17(11-12), 1365-73.

[85] Zhu L, Vranckx R, Khau Van Kien P, Lalande A, Boisset N, Mathieu F, et al. Mutations in myosin heavy chain 11 cause a syndrome associating thoracic aortic aneurysm/aortic dissection and patent ductus arteriosus. *Nature genetics*. 2006, 38(3), 343-9.

[86] Pannu, H; Tran-Fadulu, V; Papke, CL; Scherer, S; Liu, Y; Presley, C; et al. MYH11 mutations result in a distinct vascular pathology driven by insulin-like growth factor 1 and angiotensin II. *Human molecular genetics*. 2007, 16(20), 2453-62.

[87] Bellini, C; Wang, S; Milewicz, DM; Humphrey, JD. Myh11(R247C/R247C) mutations increase thoracic aorta vulnerability to intramural damage despite a general biomechanical adaptivity. *Journal of biomechanics*. 2015, 48(1), 113-21.

[88] Kuang, SQ; Kwartler, CS; Byanova, KL; Pham, J; Gong, L; Prakash, SK; et al. Rare, nonsynonymous variant in the smooth muscle-specific isoform of myosin heavy chain, MYH11, R247C, alters force generation in the aorta and phenotype of smooth muscle cells. *Circulation research*. 2012, 110(11), 1411-22.

[89] Jackson, V; Petrini, J; Caidahl, K; Eriksson, MJ; Liska, J; Eriksson, P; et al. Bicuspid aortic valve leaflet morphology in relation to aortic root morphology: a study of 300 patients undergoing open-heart surgery. *European journal of cardio-thoracic surgery: official journal of the European Association for Cardio-thoracic Surgery*. 2011, 40(3), e118-24.

[90] Mahadevia, R; Barker, AJ; Schnell, S; Entezari, P; Kansal, P; Fedak, PW; et al. Bicuspid aortic cusp fusion morphology alters aortic three-dimensional outflow patterns, wall shear stress, and expression of aortopathy. *Circulation*. 2014, 129(6), 673-82.

[91] Merritt, BA; Turin, A; Markl, M; Malaisrie, SC; McCarthy, PM; Carr, JC. Association between leaflet fusion pattern and thoracic aorta morphology in patients with bicuspid aortic valve. *Journal of magnetic resonance imaging: JMRI*. 2014, 40(2), 294-300.

[92] Schaefer, BM; Lewin, MB; Stout, KK; Gill, E; Prueitt, A; Byers, PH; et al. The bicuspid aortic valve: an integrated phenotypic classification of leaflet morphology and aortic root shape. *Heart*. 2008, 94(12), 1634-8.

[93] Vergara, C; Viscardi, F; Antiga, L; Luciani, GB. Influence of bicuspid valve geometry on ascending aortic fluid dynamics: a parametric study. *Artificial organs*. 2012, 36(4), 368-78.

[94] Chiu, JJ; Usami, S; Chien, S. Vascular endothelial responses to altered shear stress: pathologic implications for atherosclerosis. *Annals of medicine*. 2009, 41(1), 19-28.

[95] Davies, PF. Hemodynamic shear stress and the endothelium in cardiovascular pathophysiology. *Nature clinical practice Cardiovascular medicine*. 2009, 6(1), 16-26.

[96] Dekker, RJ; van, Soest, S; Fontijn, RD; Salamanca, S; de, Groot, PG; VanBavel, E; et al. Prolonged fluid shear stress induces a distinct set of endothelial cell genes, most specifically lung Kruppel-like factor (KLF2). *Blood*. 2002, 100(5), 1689-98.

[97] Hope, MD; Hope, TA; Meadows, AK; Ordovas, KG; Urbania, TH; Alley, MT; et al. Bicuspid aortic valve: four-dimensional MR evaluation of ascending aortic systolic flow patterns. *Radiology*. 2010, 255(1), 53-61.

[98] Groenendijk, BC; Hierck, BP; Gittenberger-De, Groot, AC; Poelmann, RE. Development-related changes in the expression of shear stress responsive genes KLF-2, ET-1, and NOS-3 in the developing cardiovascular system of chicken embryos. *Developmental dynamics: an official publication of the American Association of Anatomists*. 2004, 230(1), 57-68.

[99] Groenendijk, BC; Van, der, Heiden, K; Hierck, BP; Poelmann, RE. The role of shear stress on ET-1, KLF2, and NOS-3 expression in the developing cardiovascular system of chicken embryos in a venous ligation model. *Physiology*. 2007, 22, 380-9.

[100] Laforest, B; Nemer, M. GATA5 interacts with GATA4 and GATA6 in outflow tract development. *Developmental biology*. 2011, 358(2), 368-78.

[101] Liu, A; Nickerson, A; Troyer, A; Yin, X; Cary, R; Thornburg, K; et al. Quantifying blood flow and wall shear stresses in the outflow tract of chick embryonic hearts. *Computers & structures*. 2011, 89(11-12), 855-67.

[102] Barker, AJ; Markl, M; Burk, J; Lorenz, R; Bock, J; Bauer, S; et al. Bicuspid aortic valve is associated with altered wall shear stress in the

ascending aorta. *Circulation Cardiovascular imaging*. 2012, 5(4), 457-66.

[103] Bissell, MM; Hess, AT; Biasiolli, L; Glaze, SJ; Loudon, M; Pitcher, A; et al. Aortic dilation in bicuspid aortic valve disease: flow pattern is a major contributor and differs with valve fusion type. *Circulation Cardiovascular imaging*. 2013, 6(4), 499-507.

[104] Grewal, N; Gittenberger-de Groot, AC; DeRuiter, MC; Klautz, RJ; Poelmann, RE; Duim, S; et al. Bicuspid aortic valve: phosphorylation of c-Kit and downstream targets are prognostic for future aortopathy. *European journal of cardio-thoracic surgery: official journal of the European Association for Cardio-thoracic Surgery*. 2014, 46(5), 831-9.

[105] Balistreri, CR; Pisano, C; Candore, G; Maresi, E; Codispoti, M; Ruvolo, G. Focus on the unique mechanisms involved in thoracic aortic aneurysm formation in bicuspid aortic valve versus tricuspid aortic valve patients: clinical implications of a pilot study. *European journal of cardio-thoracic surgery: official journal of the European Association for Cardio-thoracic Surgery*. 2013, 43(6), e180-6.

[106] Drapisz, S; Goralczyk, T; Jamka-Miszalski, T; Olszowska, M; Undas, A. Nonstenotic bicuspid aortic valve is associated with elevated plasma asymmetric dimethylarginine. *Journal of cardiovascular medicine*. 2013, 14(6), 446-52.

[107] Maleki, S; Bjorck, HM; Folkersen, L; Nilsson, R; Renner, J; Caidahl, K; et al. Identification of a novel flow-mediated gene expression signature in patients with bicuspid aortic valve. *Journal of molecular medicine*. 2013, 91(1), 129-39.

[108] Tzemos, N; Lyseggen, E; Silversides, C; Jamorski, M; Tong, JH; Harvey, P; et al. Endothelial function, carotid-femoral stiffness, and plasma matrix metalloproteinase-2 in men with bicuspid aortic valve and dilated aorta. *Journal of the American College of Cardiology*. 2010, 55(7), 660-8.

[109] Sachdev, V; Matura, LA; Sidenko, S; Ho, VB; Arai, AE; Rosing, DR; et al. Aortic valve disease in Turner syndrome. *Journal of the American College of Cardiology*. 2008, 51(19), 1904-9.

[110] van, Engelen, K; Bartelings, MM; Gittenberger-de, Groot, AC; Baars, MJ; Postma, AV; Bijlsma, EK; et al. Bicuspid aortic valve morphology and associated cardiovascular abnormalities in fetal Turner syndrome: a pathomorphological study. *Fetal diagnosis and therapy*. 2014, 36(1), 59-68.

[111] Acharya, A; Hans, CP; Koenig, SN; Nichols, HA; Galindo, CL; Garner, HR, et al. Inhibitory role of Notch1 in calcific aortic valve disease. *PloS one*. 2011, 6(11), e27743.

[112] Foffa, I; Murzi, M; Mariani, M; Mazzone, AM; Glauber, M; Ait, Ali, L; et al. Angiotensin-converting enzyme insertion/deletion polymorphism is a risk factor for thoracic aortic aneurysm in patients with bicuspid or tricuspid aortic valves. *The Journal of thoracic and cardiovascular surgery*. 2012, 144(2), 390-5.

[113] Martin, M; Pichel, IA; Florez, Munoz, JP; Naves-Diaz, M; Palacin, M, Cannata-Andia, JB; et al. Low transcriptional activity haplotype of matrix metalloproteinase 1 is less frequent in bicuspid aortic valve patients. *Gene*. 2013, 524(2), 304-8.

[114] Pisano, C; Maresi, E; Balistreri, CR; Candore, G; Merlo, D; Fattouch, K; et al. Histological and genetic studies in patients with bicuspid aortic valve and ascending aorta complications. *Interactive cardiovascular and thoracic surgery*. 2012, 14(3), 300-6.

[115] van Rooij, E; Sutherland, LB; Thatcher, JE; DiMaio, JM; Naseem, RH, Marshall, WS; et al. Dysregulation of microRNAs after myocardial infarction reveals a role of miR-29 in cardiac fibrosis. Proceedings of the National Academy of Sciences of the United States of America. 2008, 105(35), 13027-32.

[116] Boon, RA; Seeger, T; Heydt, S; Fischer, A; Hergenreider, E; Horrevoets, AJ, et al. MicroRNA-29 in aortic dilation: implications for aneurysm formation. *Circulation research*. 2011, 109(10), 1115-9.

[117] Nishimura, RA; Otto, CM; Bonow, RO; Carabello, BA; Erwin, JP; 3rd, Guyton, RA; et al. 2014 AHA/ACC guideline for the management of patients with valvular heart disease: a report of the American College of Cardiology/American Heart Association Task Force on Practice Guidelines. *The Journal of thoracic and cardiovascular surgery*. 2014, 148(1), e1-e132.

In: Bicuspid Aortic Valve
Editor: Anthony Chapman

ISBN: 978-1-63482-786-7

Chapter 3

Genetic Basis, Pathogenesis and Histopathology of Aortopathy in Bicuspid Aortic Valve and Marfan syndrome

Junfeng Yan*[1]*, Ann-Cathrin Lehsau*[1]*,
Pamela Lazar-Karsten*[1]*, Detlev Schult-Badusche*[1]*,
Luc Mertens*[2]*, Bart L. Loeys*[3] *and Salah A. Mohamed*[1]*
[1]Department of Cardiac and Thoracic Vascular Surgery, UK SH-Campus Luebeck, Luebeck, Germany
[2]The Hospital for Sick Children, Toronto, Candada
[3]Center of Medical Genetics, University of Antwerp and University Hospital of Antwerp, Belgium, Radhoud University, Nijmegen, The Netherlands

Abstract

Aortic aneurysms are characterized by weakened aortic walls and are relatively common causes of death because of arterial dissection or rupture. The most common causes of thoracic aortic aneurysm are congenital genetic defects in the aortic wall. These can occur in association with pathological conditions such as Marfan syndrome (MFS)

* salah.mohamed@uksh.de.

and bicuspid aortic valve (BAV). Many studies have observed similarities between the histology of the aneurysmal tissue of the aorta in MFS and BAV. In MFS, mutations in the gene encoding for the extracellular matrix protein fibrillin-1 have been detected; this mutation leads to dysregulation of transforming growth factor-beta (TGF-b) signaling. In contrast, the genetics underlying BAV are largely unknown. The current grading of aortic abnormalities during histopathological evaluation of BAV is based on conflicting reports. Thus, whether mechanisms related to the existing aneurysmal histological alterations in BAV are due to genetic etiology and/or wall stress induced by flow turbulence requires further investigation. The heritability of BAV is high, estimated at 0.75–0.89. Family-based genome-wide analyses revealed a linkage between BAV and chromosomal regions 5q, 13q, and 18q in autosomal dominant inheritance with reduced penetrance and a non-Mendelian pattern.

A male predominance of more than 3:1 has been reported for BAV, and this anomaly is very frequent in X0 Turner's syndrome (incidence rate: 22–34%), suggesting an X-linked contribution. In one family with Anderson syndrome four family members were described with BAV. In Anderson syndrome, a mutation in the *potassium inwardly-rectifying channel, subfamily J, member 2* is observed. Mutations were detected in the transmembrane receptor *NOTCH1*. Moreover, mutations in the vascular smooth muscle cell alpha actin gene (*ACTA2*) have also been identified in patients with BAV and aortic aneurysms. Furthermore, BAV can manifest as part of defects in the left ventricular outflow tract spectrum including aortic coarctation, arch hypoplasia, and supravalvular and mitral valve stenosis. The *UFD1L* gene, which is highly expressed in the outflow tract during embryogenesis, is down-regulated in the cusps of patients with BAV compared with those of control patients. Heterozygous loss of *Nkx2-5*, *Fgf8*, and *GATA5* in mice predisposes for the development of BAV. Tissue-specific deletion of the gene encoding activin receptor type 1 (*Alk2/Acvr1*) in the cushion mesenchyme is observed to result in formation of aortic valve defects including BAV. Endothelial nitric oxide synthase (eNOS) is also associated with the development of BAV in mice. A high incidence of aortic aneurysms was detected in eNOS/apolipoprotein E double-knockout mice. Recent studies also reported a significant decrease in the amount of the eNOS protein present in aneurysmal BAV aortic tissue compared with tricuspid aortic valve (TAV) tissue. Local differences in eNOS protein expression were observed in BAV compared with TAV aortic aneurysms, probably due to variations in aortic wall shear stresses. Dysregulated TGF-b activity, dysregulation of miRNAs, and loss of aortic medial elastic fibers are observed in ascending aortic aneurysms and acute aortic dissection (AAD). Patients with BAV are at an increased risk of developing AAD (5 to 9 times more than normal; 12.5 to 20.5 times more than patients with MFS).

In this chapter, we review our present understanding of ascending thoracic aortic aneurysm pathogenesis. We discuss the genetic basis and basic pathology underlying BAV and ascending thoracic aortic aneurysms, and compare these to known mechanisms underlying other aortopathologies. Histopathological findings in dilated aortic walls of BAV were compared with dilated TAV and MFS.

Frequency and Possible Causes of Aortic Dilation (Aneurysms)

2.1. External and Genetic Factors

The aorta, the main artery of great body circulatory system, rises as an opening above the left ventricle, which is closed by the aortic valve (Figure 1A). A healthy aorta is an elastic vessel, and has a certain size that correlates with age and gender. The aorta is divided into five sections: the ascending part of the aortic root (aortic valve along with the sinus portion) is called ascending aorta, it ranges up to the bifurcation of the *truncus brachiocephalicus*. The aortic arch follows the ascending aorta then ends with the descending part of the aorta, which comprises the thoracic aorta and then the abdominal aorta. The normal aortic diameter in adults is approximately 35 mm. A vessel bulge (aneurysm) is defined as permanent and exceeding of the standard value involving all layers of the vessel wall (Fig. 1B). Thoracic aortic aneurysms are localized to 51% in the ascending aorta, to 38% in the descending aorta, and 11% of aneurysms can be found in the aortic arch. (Bickerstaff et al., 1982; Recklinghausen, 1855) Thoracic aortic aneurysms without treatment can by growth and rupture cause death (Fig. 1C, 1D).

A microscopic qualitative change in the aortic wall was first described in the nineteenth century in patients with aneurysms. The aneurysmal aortic wall is mainly characterized by degeneration and a reduced number of elastic fibers of the media which results in weakening of the aortic wall, and consequent dilation. Aortic aneurysms are multifactorial diseases, so several theories on the origin of the formation of the aorta have been claimed over time.

A first theory was described in 1883 by von Recklinghausen and says that a lesion of the *tunica media* is caused by mechanical operations, such as trauma, alone (Recklinghausen, 1855). Malkoff joined the theory of von Recklinghausen and studied the impact of trauma on the artery walls. To do this he squeezed them with a tweezer and he derived from the studies that traumas change the vessel wall of the arteries. It is pliable, so at this point aneurysms can form (Malkoff, 1899). A second theory, which describes a further cause of the lesion of the *tunica media*, is known under the name of 'inflammation theory' (Lichtenstein, 1901). As the name implies, inflammations are responsible for the destruction of elastic tissue and thus the weakening of the aortic wall. The innermost layer of the artery is inflamed due to infection (endarteriitis) in the *vasa vasorum*. *Vasa vasorum* supplies the *tunica adventitia* and in particular the *tunica media* with nutrients and oxygen Infectious diseases, such as syphilis, are possible causes of inflammatory foci. The inflamed *vasorum* evokes a thickening of the wall and the lumen of the *vasa vasorum* also narrows. The result is a deprivation of nutrients and oxygen in the *tunica media*, which leads to death of elastic fibres and muscle cells in this aortic layer. Inflamed areas transform into inelastic, thickened scar tissue, this process is called necrosis.

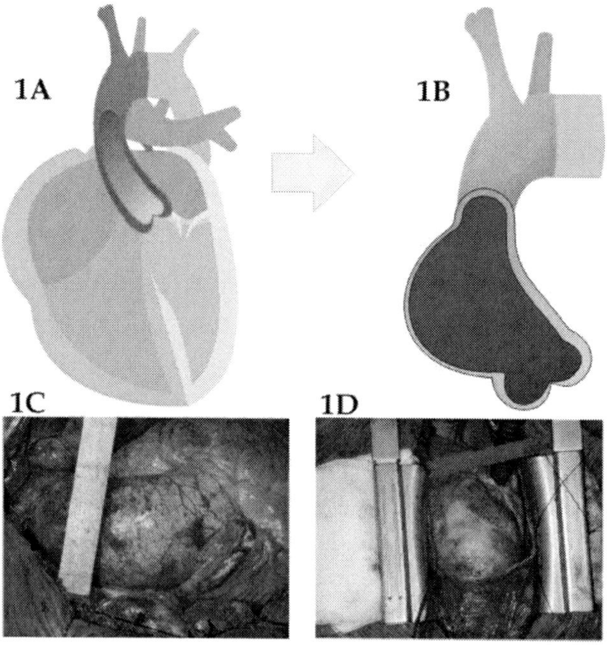

Figure 1. Schematic representation of ascending aorta in 1A; dilation of the convex aortic site in 1B; typically ectasia formations of the ascending sections (cluster II) depicted in respect to Fazel-classification in BAV-cohort in 1C; acute aortic dissection type A shown in 1D.

Thus an aneurysm is formed as inelastic aortic wall and will give in to the high blood pressure. (Nesi et al., 2009) A further theory about the origin of aneurysm formation describes atherosclerosis as the cause. (Wolpert, 1905) Pathological changes in the vessel walls are known in arteriosclerosis, which increasingly narrow the blood vessels up to complete occlusion. This process is facilitated by several risk factors, such as chronic arterial hypertension, hyperlipidemia, smoking, diabetes mellitus and aging. (Bonow et al., 2006; Hahn et al., 1992) The latter are probably more important in abdominal than in thoracic aortic aneurysm.

In addition to the described external factors, a number of genetic factors have been shown to contribute to the pathogenesis of aortic aneurysms. (Guo et al., 2001; Kroner et al., 2011)

2.1.1. Loeys-Dietz Syndrome

Loeys-Dietz syndrome (LDS) is a severe aortic aneurysm syndrome, which is characterized by vascular and skeletal manifestations. The underlying cause of the syndrome was initially shown to be mutations in the genes for the receptors TGFBR1 or TGFBR2 of the growth transforming growth factor beta (Loeys et al., 2005), but recently also mutations in SMAD3, TGFB2 and TGFB3 were shown to be involved in LDS. (Bertoli-Avella et al., 2015) TGFB is involved in cell proliferation, cell differentiation, cell migration, and tissue organization in the early stages of development. Huge aneurysms occur in Loeys-Dietz syndrome, which are not only found in the aorta, but also widely in other arteries. Patients with Loeys-Dietz syndrome are also characterized by abnormal increased distance between the eyes (orbital hypertelorism), as well as premature fusion of the skull suture (craniosynostosis), and cleft palate (*palatoschisis).* In addition, translucent skin is another characteristic of Loeys-Dietz syndrome with high vulnerability to atrophic scarring. (Dietz et al., 2005a; Loeys et al., 2006)

2.1.2. Ehlers-Danlos Syndrome

The Ehlers–Danlos syndrome includes a heterogenous group of inherited connective tissue diseases, which are classified, into different primary types: the classic, the hypermobile type or the vascular type but many other rare forms have been identified recently. These syndromes is characterized by hyperelasticity of the skin with vulnerability to atrophic scar formation, but also rupture of the arteries and internal organs such as spleen, intestines, or of the uterus. (Callewaert et al., 2008a) In contrast to the complications associated with the classical or hypermobile type, additional serious vascular complications occur in the vascular type. In the latter form, mutations in the *collagen type III alpha 1* gene (COL3A1) result in defective type III collagen synthesis associated with aneurysms in the arteries, but importantly dissection can also occur with predisposing aneurysm. (Callewaert et al., 2008a; Malfait et al., 1993)

In the classic type of Ehlers–Danlos syndrome (prior types I and II), the most common cause is molecular defects of COL5A1 and COL5A2, but also mutations in the tenascin-X and COL1A2 have been described. (Malfait et al., 2005) Half of the mutations that cause the classic Ehlers–Danlos syndrome are likely to affect the COL5A1 gene, a significant portion of mutations result in low levels of mRNA from the mutant allele as a consequence of nonsense-mediated mRNA decay. (Loeys et al., 2006; Malfait et al., 2005) The genetic basis of the hypermobile type is currently unknown.

2.1.3. Arterial Tortuosity Syndrome

Arterial tortuosity syndrome is a rare autosomal recessive connective tissue disorder. In addition to skin, skeletal and joint anomalies, this syndrome is characterized mainly by its vascular manifestation. These include stenosis and aneurysms in the aorta and in other arteries. The underlying cause of the arterial tortuosity syndrome is a mutation in the *solute carrier family 2, member 10 gene* (SLC_2A_{10}), which encodes the glucose transporter 10 (GLUT10). It was hypothesized that as a result, a reduced transcription of decorin takes place, which is a known inhibitor for TGFB (Pomianowski et al., 2013). However, in which way exactly TGFB influences the aneurysm formation, is still unclear, but its role in the vascular morphogenesis was confirmed. (Callewaert et al., 2008a; Callewaert et al., 2008b; Coucke et al., 2006)

2.1.4. Autosomal Dominant Polycystic Kidney Disease (ADPKD)

The main feature of the hereditary disorder ADPKD is a bilateral progressive increase in number and size of renal cysts, which may lead to end stage renal disease (ESRD). Approximately 85–90% of patients with ADPKD have an abnormal short arm of chromosome 16 [i.e., ADPKD type 1 (ADPKD1)]. Another defect found on the long arm of chromosome 4 results in ADPKD type 2 (ADPKD2) and is responsible for 10–15% of ADPKD cases. A third genotype may exist, but the genomic locus for the same is unknown. Proteins that are encoded by PKD1 and PKD2 i.e., polycystin 1 and polycystin 2, respectively, seem to function together to regulate the morphological configuration of epithelial cells. The polycystins are expressed during development as early as the blastocyst stage and are expressed in a broad array of terminally differentiated tissues. The functions of the polycystins in epithelial tissues of the kidney, liver, and vascular smooth muscles have been scrutinized to the greatest extent. In some patients, a combined phenotype of Marfan-like connective tissue disorder and ADPCKD has been described (Gillis et al., 2013). Patients with ADPKD can also present with hepatic cysts, cerebral vascular aneurysms, annuloaortic ectasia, and abdominal aneurysms. (Gonzalez-Perrett et al., 2001)

2.1.5. Osteogenesis Imperfecta (OI)

As an inheritable connective tissue disorder, OI shows a broad phenotypical spectrum of clinical severity ranges from dominantly inherited mild bone disease with fractures, blue sclera, and low amounts of polymeric collagen, over severe bone disease, normal colored sclera, and polymeric collagen of reduced stability to very severe bone disease in occasional infants who die at or soon after birth due to abnormal polymeric collagen. The differences are supposed to be due to distinct abnormalities of collagen metabolism. Most OI mutations are located in the N-anchor region of type I procollagen and are predominated by glycine substitution. However, recently several recessive forms of OI have also been described. (Shi et al., 2015)

2.1.6. Familial Thoracic Aortic Aneurysms and Dissections

Familial thoracic aortic aneurysm and dissection (familial TAAD) occurs in patients without detected genetic syndromes and it accounts for up to 20% of thoracic aneurysms and dissections. The occurrence and timing of these aortic abnormalities vary, even among the members of the same family with a history of the disease. They can begin in childhood or not occur until late in life. Aortic dilatation is generally the first feature of familial TAAD to develop; however, in some affected individuals, dissection occurs with little or no aortic dilation. Familial TAAD has also been associated with coarctation of the aorta, bicuspid aortic valve and aortic root dilation. Several genes and loci are known to be associated with familial TAAD (e.g. transforming growth factor beta receptor type I and receptor type II, smooth muscle-specific myosin heavy chain (*MYH11*), smooth muscle-specific alpha-actin (*ACTA2*), myosin light chain kinase (*MYLK*), mothers against decapentaplegic homolog 3 (*SMAD3*)). *MYH11* gene is mutated in families which display a phenotype of thoracic aortic aneurysms and dissections specifically paired with a patent ductus ateriosus. The *ACTA2* gene is made to be responsible for ~10%-14% of inherited ascending thoracic aortic aneurysms and dissections. (Guo et al.,

2001; Guo et al., 2009; Kroner et al., 2011; Mendoza et al., 2011; Milewicz et al., 2008; Pearson et al., 2008)

2.1.7. Turner Syndrome

Turner's syndrome (TS) occurs approximately in 1 out of 2500 live female births. The most common lesions of cardiac malformations in TS are the coarctation of the aorta and bicuspid aortic valve defect. Aortic root dilatation and hypertension have also been recognized to have an increased risk of occurrence in women with TS. Therefore, cardiovascular abnormalities are one of the main causes of increased mortality in TS, particularly during childhood. Nearly 50% of the patients presenting with TS have a pure X chromosome monosomy (45, X0), the other 50% show mosaics, which are characterized by other X chromosome aberrations, such as [45,X0/46,XX; 45,X0/46,X,i(Xq); 45,X0/46,X,r(X)]. (Elsheikh et al., 2001; Lippe1991; Sybert et al., 2004) Additionally, abnormalities and mosaicism with Y chromosome (e.g., 45,X0/46,XY) are also present. Patients with TS have a highly increased risk of congenital cardiovascular anomalies and most reports conclude that echocardiographic evaluation is essential after the diagnosis of TS. (Mazzanti et al., 1998) Additionally, abnormalities and mosaicism with Y chromosome (e.g., 45,X0/46,XY) have also been described. (Partsch et al., 1994)

2.1.8. Marfan Syndrome

Marfan syndrome (MFS) was named after Antoine Marfan, a French pediatrician. MFS is characterized by distinctive skeletal changes: disproportionately long limbs, narrow fingers, tall stature, abnormal joints flexibilty, scoliosis, and chest wall deformities, such as a funnel or pigeon chest. Other important features include ectopia lentis, or other retinal detachment, mitral valve prolapse, pneumothorax and hernias. However, aortic aneurysm rupture constitutes the most lethal manifestation that reduces life expectancy to only 32-35 years if untreated. As such, MFS is a pleiotropic disorder involving a variety of organ systems. However, not every patient diagnosed with Marfan's syndrome is affected with all above mentioned organ diseases, hampering a clinical diagnosis of MFS. MFS is an autosomal dominant inherited disease of the extracellular connective tissue that can occur also as the result of a de novo mutation (circa one third of patients). Regardless of gender, MFS is diagnosed with a frequency of 1/3000 to 1/5000. (Abraham et al., 1982; Boileau et al., 1993; De et al., 1996; Dietz et al., 1994)

The genetic cause of MFS is mutations in the FBN1 gene (encoding for fibrillin-1) on chromosome 15. Fibrillin is a glycoprotein, which is present in the microfibrils of the extracellular matrix in the connective tissue. Both Fibrillin-1 and Fibrillin-2 contribute together with tropoelastin and other glycoproteins to the formation of elastic fibers and determine in this way to the train elasticity of tissue. Microfibrils exist everywhere in the body, where the mechanical stress is high even without association to elastin (e.g. in the ciliary muscle of the eye). Fibrillin-1 is characterized by special cysteine-rich structures, called EGF domains (epidermal growth factor domains). Most of the EGF-like regions bind calcium. Calcium occupies a key role in the folding of fibrillins and thus contributes to a stable and a compact structure of the Fibrillin. In this structure, Fibrillin-1 is protected against proteolysis by enzymes such as metalloproteinase. (Sakai et al., 1986)

The discovery of Fibrillins contributes to the understanding of molecular genetic causes of MFS, realized by Dietz in 1991 in the Johns Hopkins University in Baltimore. He found together with his group, that a first mutation in the *fibrillin-1* gene (*FBN1*), located on the long arm of chromosome 15 (15q15-q21.1) leads to structural changes and this cause the complex diseases of many different body organs. Different point mutations can occur, such as insertions, deletions or duplications due to splicing errors, which lead to a wrong read of frame shifts of the DNA substitutions. Missense mutations can alter amino acids in 1 of 47 EGF-like domains. EGF-like domains are predicted to bind calcium based on a conserved consensus sequence for calcium binding. (De et al., 1996; Dietz et al., 1991; Dietz1993; Dietz et al., 1995; Dietz1995; Dietz et al., 2005b)

Role of TGFbeta Signaling in MFS

Today it is accepted that FBN-1 mutations serve as triggers for secondary processes with strong impact on the expression of characteristic Marfan syndrome symptoms and transforming growth factor-beta (TGFB) playing a pivotal role. (Robinson et al., 2006) TGFB is a pleiotropic cytokine of compact structure with 4 B-sheets stabilized by three intramolecular disulfide-bridges. Due to this structural property TGFB can only arduously be denatured and therefore is very suitable as extracellular signal protein. Depending on cell type and the target cell`s stage of development TGFB shows diverse activities by binding to TGFB receptors in the cell membrane. (ten et al., 2004) There are various TGFB receptors. The main receptor is a heterodimer transmembrane protein of receptor type I and II containing an intrinsic Serin-Threonin-kinase regulating signal transduction. Stimulated by TGFB, the

TGFB receptors activate phosphorylation of SMAD2 and SMAD3 proteins which migrate into the nucleus as a heterodimer complex with SMAD4 Here the complex binds to DNA and by this regulates gene transcription. TGFB activity is determined by latent TGFB-binding proteins (LTBP). In addition to structural functions in the extracellular matrix LTBP serve to bind TGFB via latency associated peptides (LAP). Notably LTBP-1, LTBP-3 and LTBP-4 execute this double-function. In this process LTBP are in close association with FBN-1, a fact representing an important aspect in research on the pathogenesis of the Marfan syndrome. (Neptune et al., 2003; Robinson et al., 2006) Substitutions in *FBN-1* therefore not only result in reduced parts of Cysteine- and Calcium-ligands, but also impair FBN-1 and LTBP association capabilities. A respective lower amount of TGFB can be bound with the effect of a large part of these proteins remaining unbound in the extracellular matrix causing hyperactivity of the TGFB signaling pathway.

The relation between the TGFB signaling pathway and Marfan syndrome disorders is not yet clarified. There are however promising suggestions to explain this relation. It is hypothesized that hyperactivity of the TGFB signaling pathway induces more metalloproteases to destroy fibrillin structures by proteolysis and thereby increase aortic wall attenuation. In addition Fibrillin-1 fragments cleaved by proteolysis potentially stimulate further metalloproteases. It is also assumed that metalloproteases activate the immune response leading to aortic wall infiltration by T-lymphocytes and monocytes/macrophages. This process evokes aortic wall inflammation. Thickened and rigid cicatricial tissue results from inflammation and represents a basic condition for the development of aortic aneurysms. (Robinson et al., 2006) These assumptions still have to be confirmed, however a significantly elevated level of free TGFB and metalloproteases as well as increased Smad-protein phosphorylation could already been shown in aortas showing aneurysm formation. (Habashi et al., 2006) Although correlations still have to be clarified these results constitute a major progress in research on the pathogenesis of MFS.

2.1.9. Bicuspid Aortic Valve

Bicuspid aortic valve (BAV) is the most common of the congenital cardiac malformations with an estimated incidence of 1-2% in the general population. (Roberts1970) BAV has a high heritability of ≈ 0.89. A family-based genome-wide analysis found that BAV was linked to chromosomal regions 5q, 13q, and 18q with autosomal dominant inheritance, reduced penetrance, and a non-Mendelian pattern. (Cripe et al., 2004; Huntington et al., 1997; Ward2000) Mutations have been detected in the transmembrane receptor *NOTCH1* (gene map locus 9q) in familial and sporadic BAV cases. (Garg et al., 2005; Mohamed et al., 2006) Mutations in the *vascular smooth muscle cell alpha actin* gene (mapped to chromosome 10q) have also been identified in BAV patients. (Guo et al., 2009) Downregulated expression of *ubiquitin fusion degradation 1-like*, a gene that is highly expressed in the outflow tract during embryogenesis, was observed in the cusps of BAV patients as compared with those of controls. (Mohamed et al., 2005) Heterozygous *Nkx2-5*-deficient, *Fgf8*, and *Gata5* mice are at higher risks for developing BAV. Tissue-specific deletion of the gene, that encodes for the activin receptor type 1 (*Alk2/Acvr1*) in the cushion mesenchyme results in the formation of aortic valve defects, including BAV. In mice, endothelial nitric oxide synthase (eNOS) is also associated with the development of BAV. BAV can also manifest as different types of left ventricular outflow tract abnormalities, including aortic coarctation, arch hypoplasia, and supravalvular and mitral valve stenosis. (Laforest et al., 2011; Lee et al., 2000; Macatee et al., 2003; Schott et al., 1998; Wessels et al., 2005) A male predominance of more than 3:1 has been reported for BAV, and this anomaly is very frequent in X0 Turner's syndrome (incidence rate: 22–34%), suggesting an X-linked etiology. An analysis of a subpopulation with Anderson syndrome described 4 members with BAV. In Andersen's syndrome, there is a mutation in the *potassium inwardly-rectifying channel, subfamily J, member 2* (*KCNJ2*) gene. (Andelfinger et al., 2002; Miller et al., 1983) A genome-wide association study applying gene network analysis techniques identified some haplotypes that were associated with BAV *AXIN1/PDIA2* and *endoglin*. (Wooten et al., 2010) Proteomic studies observed the association of HSP27 and four phosphoproteins with BAV. (Matt et al., 2007) Recent studies observed the involvement of microRNAs (miRNAs) in BAV disease. MiRNAs are small, approximately 22 nucleotides in length noncoding nucleotide RNAs, and have been shown to modulate mRNA stability and translation. (Cordes et al., 2009; van et al., 2007a; van et al., 2007b) Nigam et al. demonstrated that miR-26a was down-regulated in fused aortic valve. (Nigam et al., 2010) The miR-26a was also found to be down-regulated in aneurysms. (Leeper et al., 2011) However, the exact genetic cause of BAV remains unknown. Though, BAV not only contributes considerably to cardiovascular health risks but also represents a technical challenge in cardiac valve operations. More than 50% of patients with BAV also suffer from a dilation of the ascending aorta.

Histopathological findings in dilated aortic walls of BAV are also very complex. Early studies report cystic media necrosis, elastin fragmentation as well as loss of smooth muscle cells and their orientation in aneurysmal aortic walls. (Fedak et al., 2005) Other studies show evidence of less aneurysmal aortic wall modifications in BAV patients compared to those of TAV patients. Furthermore it could be shown that the elastic membrane of aneurysmal aortas in BAV patients is thinner than that of TAV patients and that the distance between the single elastic lamellae increases in correlation with increasing aorta diameters. These diverse findings hint at the complexity of dilation of the ascending aorta associated with BAV aortopathy. While the pathogenesis of aneurysm in patients with connective tissue disorders, such as Marfan syndrome, is better understood, the emergence of thoracic aneurysm in patients with BAV is still unclear. Recent studies examined two components of the TGFB pathway, TGFB and pSMAD2, involved in vascular remodeling. TGFB expression spread out from the intima to the inner media. The findings suggest that there is no inherent difference between BAV and TAV with respect to TGFß signaling. Instead, the bioavailability and effects of active TGFB are muted in patients with BAV as is the expression of Endoglin, a type III auxiliary receptor for the TGFB superfamily. (Grewal *et.al.* 2014, Paloschi *et. al.* 2015, Kapur *et. al.* 2013) It is controversial whether in patients with onset dilation of the ascending aorta, sections of the aorta during an aortic valve operation also need to be replaced.

3. Matrix Metalloproteinase Expression in the Aortopathy of the Ascending Aorta

Present knowledge of the aortopathy (aneurysms) in patients with BAV reflects only a part of the complex pathogenesis. (Mohamed and Sievers, 2011) Aortic aneurysms are multifactor diseases, so several theories on the origin of aortic formation have been proposed over time. Cellular and extracellular processes are involved in the pathogenesis of ascending thoracic aneurysms in patients with BAV. Elevation of matrix metalloproteinases (MMPs) achieved by aortic aneurysms has long been recognized. (Hahn et al., 1992; Roberts1970) However, current knowledge of matrix protein expression in aneurysmal tissues of aortic abnormalities of the ascending aorta is based on conflicting reports. Thus, whether mechanisms related to existing aneurysmal histological alterations in BAV are due to genetic heterotopy and/or wall stress induced by flow turbulence requires further investigation. BAV is associated with thoracic ascending aneurysms (TAA) that can lead to acute aortic dissection, which is a life-threatening condition with high morbidity and mortality rates and is generally an unpredictable event. There are various reports in the literature on matrix protein expression in aneurysmal tissues. On the basis of the published data, research on abdominal aortic aneurysm (AAA) began considerably earlier than research on TAA. Some aspects of AAA research allow conclusions to be drawn about TAA, whereas in other regards, the following differences have been recognized. It is known that MMPs and tissue inhibitors of metalloproteinases (TIMPs) have crucial roles in the development of AAA. Inflammatory AAA mainly involves an increase in detectable MMP-9, while mouse models have also shown an elevation of MMP-12. Both are secreted by macrophages. An increase in MMP-2 secretion has been observed in smooth muscle cells and fibroblasts in an animal model. In recent years, several insights into TAA have become known. MMP-2 levels are elevated in almost all studies concerning BAV-associated aneurysms compared with the levels of TAV-associated TAAs. The findings on MMP-9 have been divergent. Increased MMP-9 levels were measured in most cases, but equal levels of MMP-9 were also detected in BAV- and TAV-associated aneurysms. On the other hand, the expression of TIMPs was found to be on an equal level in BAV- and TAV-associated TAA. Different MMP/TIMP ratios have resulted from the measurement of MMP expression, whereas values >1 hinted at a proteolytic state of the aortic wall. However, a gene expression analysis of *MMP-1*, *-2,* and *-9* and of *TIMP-1* and *-2* showed no differences. This circumstance was explained by Matt et al., as resulting from differences between gene and protein expression. Their proteomic analysis showed a strong correlation between BAV- and TAV-associated aneurysms, which was considered to be an indication of pending intrinsic defects of the aortic wall. (Matt2008) We used a simultaneous detection system to acquire data on the profiles of six MMPs and their four inhibitors at four different aortic sites (concave, convex, distal, and proximal) of ascending aortic aneurysms. MMP-2, MMP-8, MMP-9, TIMP-1, TIMP-2, TIMP-3, and TIMP-4 were detected and quantified. However, protein concentrations of MMP-12 and -13 were very low. This method is as accurate as older methods and minimizes errors that can occur when measuring mRNA level using PCR techniques. (Mohamed et al., 2012a)

In a recent publication, Jackson and colleagues presented interesting results on the elevation of MMP-14 and -19 associated with TAV thoracic aortic aneurysms. They demonstrated up-regulation of MMP-14 and -19 in the media of dilated aortas. (Jackson et al., 2012) Of note, MMP-19 was the only MMP that was found to be upregulated in acute aortic dissection. (Mohamed et al., 2009) The authors have used the exon array to analyze 23 MMPs and their four inhibitors. Using these techniques with following confirmation on protein may enhance our understanding of the involvement of MMPs/TIMPs in ascending aortic aneurysms and the link to acute aortic dissection.

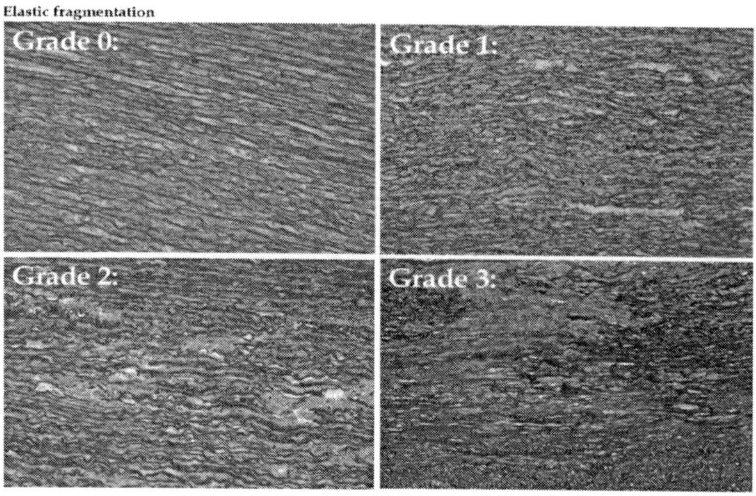

Figure 2. Histopathological evaluation, sections were studied with Verhoeff's-Van Gieson method for demonstration of elastic fibers, the grading 0 to 3 showing the fragmentation of the elastic fibers of the proximal aneurysmal ascending aorta.

4. Histopathology in the aortopathy of BAV compared to TAV and MFS dilated ascending aorta

The current grading for aortic abnormalities in histopathological evaluation is based on conflicting reports. Using the grading system according de SA et al. (Figure 2), here unexpectedly we detected differences results with respect to the dilated aortic wall changes i.e. more severe aortic wall abnormalities in TAV than in BAV patients. (de et al., 1999) In the concavity, TAV patients showed significantly higher grading of atherosclerosis, medionecrosis, cystic medial necrosis, smooth muscle cell orientation, and elastic fragmentation. Grading of atherosclerosis and smooth muscle cell orientation revealed a more severe stage in TAV distal aorta than that in BAV distal aorta, whereas the TAV convexity showed a significantly higher grading of fibrosis, atherosclerosis, medionecrosis, and smooth muscle cell orientation. TAV proximal aorta featured more severe fibrosis, atherosclerosis and medionecrosis than its BAV counterpart. Elastic fragmentation in the distal and convex aortic site of BAV correlated with the aortic diameter independent of age (data published elsewhere). These results however go in line with previous observations of our group and by Bechtel et al. (Matthias Bechtel et al., 2003) Other groups report on the difficulties of capturing all these different parameters. (Roberts et al., 2011) Therefore, we schematically show 3 parameters of proximal, convex aortic site in patients with BAV and TAV and compared them with histopathological features examined in the aortic root of Marfan syndrome patients (Figure 3).

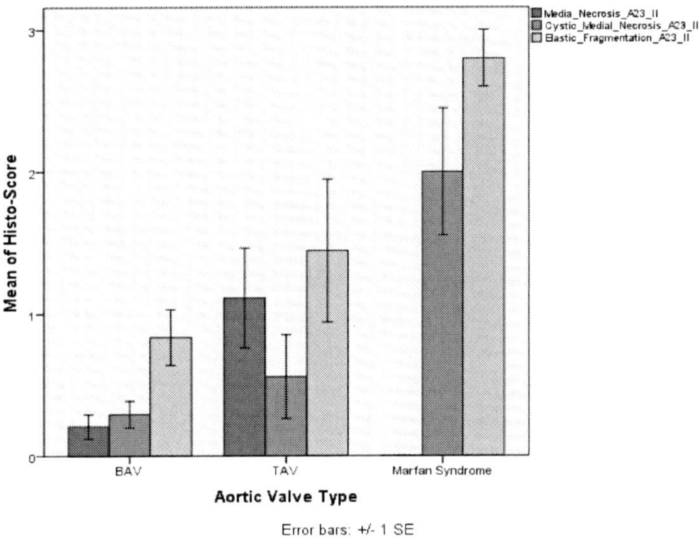

Figure 3. Comparison of histological scores was performed in terms of media necrosis, cystic media necrosis, and elastic fragmentation in the sinus section of ascending aorta aneurysms obtained from intra-operative biopsies: Aneurysms in the BAV- group demonstrated mild changes in the media with up to incipient moderate ones, while these changes were found as far as much moderate, which emphasized the presence of elastic fragmentation and cystic medial necrosis in the Marfan's syndrome group. There was a significant difference in the histological scores in terms of elastic fragmentation between the groups of TAV (M = 1.44, SEM = 1.51) and MFS (M = 2.80, SEM = 0.45), t (10.22) (p = 0.031) and highly significant difference between groups of BAV (M = 0.83, SEM = 0.96) and MFS t (27) = -4.42 (p < 0.001); whereas there was no significant difference when comparing the groups of BAV and TAV, t (10.54) = -1.13, p=0.283. Therefore, Marfan's syndrome group presents considerable stages of typical aneurysm formation. (10.54) = -1.13, p=0.283. Therefore, Marfan's syndrome group presents considerable stages of typical aneurysm formation.

Discussion

There are many syndromes associated with dilation of the ascending aorta. While the pathogenesis of aneurysm in patients with connective tissue disorders, such as Marfan-syndrome (MFS), is better understood; the emergence of thoracic aneurysm in patients with bicuspid aortic valve (BAV) is still unclear. It is controversial whether in patients with onset dilatation of the ascending aorta, sections of the aorta during an aortic valve operation also need to be replaced. This question is difficult to be answered without systematic investigation. Therefore, it is important to intensify research on aneurysm pathogenesis particularly in patients without well-known connective tissue disorders. In MFS patients, detecting the mutations in the gene encoding for the ECM protein fibrillin-1 might facilitate diagnosis and treatment (Dietz et al., 2005c; Milewicz et al., 2005). In patients with BAV, the situation is different because hemodynamics can also play a role and mutations in genes are sparely detected. The first genetic determination of BAV was described in a subpopulation of Anderson syndrome. Anderson syndrome is represented by ventricular arrhythmias, periodic scoliosis, dysmorphic features, cleft palate, and paralysis. Analysis of a large pedigree with Anderson syndrome detected 4 members (4/41) with BAV. *Potassium inwardly-rectifying channel, subfamily J, member 2* (*KCNJ2*; mapped to chromosome 17q) belongs to a large family (KCN family) of genes that produce potassium channels. The KCNJ2 gene encodes for the Kir 2.1 protein. Mutation in the *KCNJ2* gene leads to a potassium channel abnormality in Anderson syndrome. However, mechanisms by which altered potassium signaling leads to aortic valve malformations remain unknown. There is, however, a controversial debate on the etiology of BAV and BAV-associated aortopathy, not only because of the gap of knowledge on BAV anomaly, but also the heterogeneity of BAV itself (Stenosis/ regurgitation) and BAV-associated aortopathy (Fazel-Stanford clusters I, II, III, IV). (Fazel et al., 2008; Kari et al., 2012) Heritability of BAV and the coherence of gene mutations such as *Notch1, ACTA2, and GATA5* with BAV calcification and aortic dilatation seem to support a "genetic thesis." On the other hand, hemodynamic factors such as mechanical stress caused by abnormal valve anatomy have been shown to play a role in secondary valvulopathy and aortopathy. There is a correlation between eccentric BAV orifice jet aortic dilatation in wall regions prone to shear stress overload and increased formation of calcified nodules on the fused BAV leaflet. Barker et al., showed that aortic wall shear stress differs locally between BAV and control patients when examined via magnetic resonance imaging. (Barker et al., 2010) Elevation of asymmetric protein expression of matrixmetalloproteinases is researched in dilation of the ascending aorta. (Ikonomidis et al., 2007; Koullias et al., 2004; Lemaire et al., 2005; Mohamed et al., 2012a) Well documented similarities of structural changes in aneurysmal formation of the ascending aorta in BAV and MFS demonstrated how the programmed cell death (apoptosis) proceeds in smooth muscle cells (VSMC) of the aorta. (Bonderman et al., 1999; Della et al., 2008; Mohamed et al., 2010; Nataatmadja et al., 2003) Growth behaviour morphology of fractionated VSMC, and in vitro inhibition of apoptosis pathways via a caspase-3 block was investigated in vitro. (Mohamed et al., 2010) Increased presence of mitochondrial proteins in the cytosol after L-NAME treatment indicates an inhibitory effect of eNOS produced NO on the intrinsic apoptosis pathway. (Mohamed et al., 2012b) It has been demonstrated that patients with BAV suffer from more severe aortic wall abnormalities than TAV patients. Recent studies by Grewal et al., report distinct VSMC differentiation in dilated versus non-dilated and BAV versus TAV aortic walls leading to significant differences in tissue structure and maturation. The TAV aorta shows more aspects of aging. Using differentiation markers of contractile VSMCs such as smoothelin, a specific marker of highly differentiated VSMC, less maturation in BAV compared with TAV (in both dilated and non-dilated) could be detected. Smoothelin levels were significantly lower in the dilated compared with those in the non-dilated TAV aortic wall and nearly absent in all BAV specimens. (Grewal et al., 2014b) The BAV aortic wall also presented a thinner intima and less inflammation as well as decreased expressions of alpha smooth muscle actin, SM22 alpha, calponin, and lamin A/C. Lamin A/C being regulated by mechanic stress influencing vessel wall gene expression. (Swift et al., 2013) Though, the exact function of lamin A/C is not yet completely elucidated, however, it is interesting that the same group of Grewal et al., analysed further tissue of dilated BAV compared with non-dilated BAV. They detected comparable marked expression of c-Kit, phosphorylated-c-Kit, and HIF1, in dilated BAV- group and in a subgroup of the non-dilated BAV. However, the remainder of the non-dilated BAV group was significantly distinct. This difference between the dilated and non-dilated BAV was apparent for expression of the vascular remodeling factors studied. (Grewal et al., 2014a) These studies listed provide fundamental new knowledge to the pathogenesis of BAV, and with BAV associated dilation of the ascending aorta.

Conclusion and Future Directions

The question of genes or flow in the aortopathy of the ascending aorta should be considered together. There is logical causality between aortopathy and aortic valve vitien. Generally, aortic valve stenosis causes alteration in the flow dynamics leading to changed shear forces over the poststenosis aortic parts. These altered dynamics result in ectasia formations in the next aortic sections after a while. Similar phenomenon could also be observed in instances of aortic valve insufficiency. The aortic dilation in different sections is initialized by varied linear characteristics of blood flow. Furthermore, the force action between discrete aortic valve vitien and aortic ectasia is mutual, meaning that the shifts in the framework of the aorta act in deterioration of aortic valve motion characters. The vulnerability of aortic sections was mostly assessed in aortic root, aortic sinuses, sinotubular junction and ascending aorta. These could be predisposed in sense of diseases of the connective tissue. The normal dimensional distribution in distinct ascending aorta sections is impaired. A logical geometrical ratio of special ascendens parts in case of disturbed hemodynamics could facilitate therapeutic epicrisis before operative interventions, regarding postoperative prognosis.

The options of appropriate decision in different treatments for patients are debated since years. According to this, several research groups introduced some kind of related classification for clinical interests. But many of those could not basically resolve ongoing difficulties in the therapy planning. Pioneer studies showed that the pathogenesis mechanisms of aneurysmal disease also have strong similarities with the development of carcinomas and metastases. (Lindsay et al., 2011) More detailed studies of these mechanisms will therefore not only very interesting but also have promising potential for improvement in surgical intervention. Proteome analysis and new methods at the molecular level such as the matrix-assisted laser desorption/ ionization imaging mass spectrometry can provide new insights via systematic structure analysis of the affected aortic tissue in relation with histological methods.

Acknowledgments

The authors would like to acknowledge and thank the Leducq Fondation for supporting our work and giving us the opportunity to study BAV aortopathy over the coming years.

References

Abraham, P. A., Perejda, A. J., Carnes, W. H., and Uitto, J. (1982). Marfan syndrome. Demonstration of abnormal elastin in aorta. *J.Clin.Invest.*, 70(6):1245-1252.

Andelfinger, G., Tapper, A. R., Welch, R. C., Vanoye, C. G., George, A. L., Jr., and Benson, D. W. (2002). KCNJ2 mutation results in Andersen syndrome with sex-specific cardiac and skeletal muscle phenotypes. *Am.J.Hum.Genet.*, 71(3):663-668.

Barker, A. J., Lanning, C., and Shandas, R. (2010). Quantification of hemodynamic wall shear stress in patients with bicuspid aortic valve using phase-contrast MRI. *Ann.Biomed.Eng.*, 38(3):788-800.

Bertoli-Avella, A. M., Gillis, E., Morisaki, H., Verhagen, J. M., de Graaf, B. M., van de Beek, G., Gallo, E., Kruithof, B. P., Venselaar, H., Myers, L. A., Laga, S., Doyle, A. J., Oswald, G., van Cappellen, G. W., Yamanaka, I., van der Helm, R. M., Beverloo, B., de, Klein A., Pardo, L., Lammens, M., Evers, C., Devriendt, K., Dumoulein, M., Timmermans, J., Bruggenwirth, H. T., Verheijen, F., Rodrigus, I., Baynam, G., Kempers, M., Saenen, J., Van Craenenbroeck, E. M., Minatoya, K., Matsukawa, R., Tsukube, T., Kubo, N., Hofstra, R., Goumans, M. J., Bekkers, J. A., Roos-Hesselink, J. W., van de Laar, I. M., Dietz, H. C., Van, Laer L., Morisaki, T., Wessels, M. W., and Loeys, B. L. (2015). Mutations in a TGF-beta Ligand, TGFB3, Cause Syndromic Aortic Aneurysms and Dissections. *J.Am.Coll.Cardiol.*, 65(13):1324-1336.

Bickerstaff, L. K., Pairolero, P. C., Hollier, L. H., Melton, L. J., Van Peenen, H. J., Cherry, K. J., Joyce, J. W., and Lie, J. T. (1982). Thoracic aortic aneurysms: a population-based study. *Surgery.*, 92(6):1103-1108.

Boileau, C., Jondeau, G., Babron, M. C., Coulon, M., Alexandre, J. A., Sakai, L., Melki, J., Delorme, G., Dubourg, O., Bonaiti-Pellie, C., and . (1993). Autosomal dominant Marfan-like connective-tissue disorder with aortic dilation and skeletal anomalies not linked to the fibrillin genes. *Am.J.Hum.Genet.*, 53(1):46-54.

Bonderman, D., Gharehbaghi-Schnell, E., Wollenek, G., Maurer, G., Baumgartner, H., and Lang, I. M. (1999). Mechanisms underlying aortic dilatation in congenital aortic valve malformation. *Circulation.*, 99(16):2138-2143.

Bonow, R. O., Carabello, B. A., Kanu, C., de, Leon AC, Jr., Faxon, D. P., Freed, M. D., Gaasch, W. H., Lytle, B. W., Nishimura, R. A., O'Gara, P. T., O'Rourke, R. A., Otto, C. M., Shah, P. M., Shanewise, J. S., Smith, S.

C., Jr., Jacobs, A. K., Adams, C. D., Anderson, J. L., Antman, E. M., Faxon, D. P., Fuster, V., Halperin, J. L., Hiratzka, L. F., Hunt, S. A., Lytle, B. W., Nishimura, R., Page, R. L., and Riegel, B. (2006). ACC/AHA 2006 guidelines for the management of patients with valvular heart disease: a report of the American College of Cardiology/American Heart Association Task Force on Practice Guidelines (writing committee to revise the 1998 Guidelines for the Management of Patients With Valvular Heart Disease): developed in collaboration with the Society of Cardiovascular Anesthesiologists: endorsed by the Society for Cardiovascular Angiography and Interventions and the Society of Thoracic Surgeons. *Circulation.*, 114(5):e84-231.

Callewaert, B., Malfait, F., Loeys, B., and De, Paepe A. (2008a). Ehlers-Danlos syndromes and Marfan syndrome. *Best.Pract.Res.Clin.Rheumatol.*, 22(1):165-189.

Callewaert, B. L., Willaert, A., Kerstjens-Frederikse, W. S., De, Backer J., Devriendt, K., Albrecht, B., Ramos-Arroyo, M. A., Doco-Fenzy, M., Hennekam, R. C., Pyeritz, R. E., Krogmann, O. N., Gillessen-Kaesbach, G., Wakeling, E. L., Nik-zainal, S., Francannet, C., Mauran, P., Booth, C., Barrow, M., Dekens, R., Loeys, B. L., Coucke, P. J., and De Paepe, A. M. (2008b). Arterial tortuosity syndrome: clinical and molecular findings in 12 newly identified families. *Hum.Mutat.*, 29(1):150-158.

Cordes, K. R. and Srivastava, D. (2009). MicroRNA regulation of cardiovascular development. *Circ.Res.*, 104(6):724-732.

Coucke, P. J., Willaert, A., Wessels, M. W., Callewaert, B., Zoppi, N., De, Backer J., Fox, J. E., Mancini, G. M., Kambouris, M., Gardella, R., Facchetti, F., Willems, P. J., Forsyth, R., Dietz, H. C., Barlati, S., Colombi, M., Loeys, B., and De, Paepe A. (2006). Mutations in the facilitative glucose transporter GLUT10 alter angiogenesis and cause arterial tortuosity syndrome. *Nat.Genet.*, 38(4):452-457.

Cripe, L., Andelfinger, G., Martin, L. J., Shooner, K., and Benson, D. W. (2004). Bicuspid aortic valve is heritable. *J.Am.Coll.Cardiol.*, 44(1):138-143.

De, Paepe A., Devereux, R. B., Dietz, H. C., Hennekam, R. C., and Pyeritz, R. E. (1996). Revised diagnostic criteria for the Marfan syndrome. *Am.J.Med.Genet.*, 62(4):417-426.

de, Sa M., Moshkovitz, Y., Butany, J., and David, T. E. (1999). Histologic abnormalities of the ascending aorta and pulmonary trunk in patients with bicuspid aortic valve disease: clinical relevance to the ross procedure. *J.Thorac Cardiovasc Surg.*, 118(4):588-594.

Della, Corte A., Quarto, C., Bancone, C., Castaldo, C., Di, Meglio F., Nurzynska, D., De Santo, L. S., De, Feo M., Scardone, M., Montagnani, S., and Cotrufo, M. (2008). Spatiotemporal patterns of smooth muscle cell changes in ascending aortic dilatation with bicuspid and tricuspid aortic valve stenosis: focus on cell-matrix signaling. *J.Thorac Cardiovasc Surg.*, 135(1):8-18, 18.

Dietz, H. C. (1993). Marfan Syndrome.

Dietz, H. C. (1995). New insights into the genetic basis of aortic aneurysms. *Monogr Pathol.*, 37:144-155.

Dietz, H. C., Cutting, G. R., Pyeritz, R. E., Maslen, C. L., Sakai, L. Y., Corson, G. M., Puffenberger, E. G., Hamosh, A., Nanthakumar, E. J., Curristin, S. M., and . (1991). Marfan syndrome caused by a recurrent de novo missense mutation in the fibrillin gene. *Nature.*, 352(6333):337-339.

Dietz, H. C., Loeys, B., Carta, L., and Ramirez, F. (2005a). Recent progress towards a molecular understanding of Marfan syndrome. *Am.J.Med.Genet.C.Semin.Med.Genet.*, 139C(1):4-9.

Dietz, H. C., Loeys, B., Carta, L., and Ramirez, F. (2005b). Recent progress towards a molecular understanding of Marfan syndrome. *Am.J.Med.Genet.C.Semin.Med.Genet.*, 139C(1):4-9.

Dietz, H. C., Loeys, B., Carta, L., and Ramirez, F. (2005c). Recent progress towards a molecular understanding of Marfan syndrome. *Am.J.Med.Genet.C.Semin.Med.Genet.*, 139C(1):4-9.

Dietz, H. C. and Pyeritz, R. E. (1995). Mutations in the human gene for fibrillin-1 (FBN1) in the Marfan syndrome and related disorders. *Hum.Mol.Genet.*, 4 Spec No:1799-1809.

Dietz, H. C., Ramirez, F., and Sakai, L. Y. (1994). Marfan's syndrome and other microfibrillar diseases. *Adv.Hum.Genet.*, 22:153-186.

Elsheikh, M., Casadei, B., Conway, G. S., and Wass, J. A. (2001). Hypertension is a major risk factor for aortic root dilatation in women with Turner's syndrome. *Clin.Endocrinol.(Oxf).*, 54(1):69-73.

Fazel, S. S., Mallidi, H. R., Lee, R. S., Sheehan, M. P., Liang, D., Fleischman, D., Herfkens, R., Mitchell, R. S., and Miller, D. C. (2008). The aortopathy of bicuspid aortic valve disease has distinctive patterns and usually involves the transverse aortic arch. *J.Thorac.Cardiovasc.Surg.*, 135(4):901-7, 907.

Fedak, P. W., David, T. E., Borger, M., Verma, S., Butany, J., and Weisel, R. D. (2005). Bicuspid aortic valve disease: recent insights in pathophysiology and treatment. *Expert.Rev.Cardiovasc.Ther.*, 3(2):295-308.

Garg, V., Muth, A. N., Ransom, J. F., Schluterman, M. K., Barnes, R., King, I. N., Grossfeld, P. D., and Srivastava, D. (2005). Mutations in NOTCH1 cause aortic valve disease. *Nature.*, 437(7056):270-274.

Gillis, E., Van, Laer L., and Loeys, B. L. (2013). Genetics of thoracic aortic aneurysm: at the crossroad of transforming growth factor-beta signaling and vascular smooth muscle cell contractility. *Circ.Res.*, 113(3):327-340.

Gonzalez-Perrett, S., Kim, K., Ibarra, C., Damiano, A. E., Zotta, E., Batelli, M., Harris, P. C., Reisin, I. L., Arnaout, M. A., and Cantiello, H. F. (2001). Polycystin-2, the protein mutated in autosomal dominant polycystic kidney disease (ADPKD), is a Ca2+-permeable nonselective cation channel. *Proc.Natl.Acad.Sci.U.S.A.*, 98(3):1182-1187.

Grewal, N., Gittenberger-de Groot, A. C., Deruiter, M. C., Klautz, R. J., Poelmann, R. E., Duim, S., Lindeman, J. H., Koenraadt, W. M., Jongbloed, M. R., Mohamed, S. A., Sievers, H. H., Bogers, A. J., and Goumans, M. J. (2014a). Bicuspid aortic valve: phosphorylation of c-Kit and downstream targets are prognostic for future aortopathy. *Eur.J.Cardiothorac.Surg.*, 46(5):831-839.

Grewal, N., Gittenberger-de Groot, A. C., Poelmann, R. E., Klautz, R. J., Lindeman, J. H., Goumans, M. J., Palmen, M., Mohamed, S. A., Sievers, H. H., Bogers, A. J., and Deruiter, M. C. (2014b). Ascending aorta dilation in association with bicuspid aortic valve: A maturation defect of the aortic wall. *J.Thorac.Cardiovasc.Surg.*,

Guo, D., Hasham, S., Kuang, S. Q., Vaughan, C. J., Boerwinkle, E., Chen, H., Abuelo, D., Dietz, H. C., Basson, C. T., Shete, S. S., and Milewicz, D. M. (2001). Familial thoracic aortic aneurysms and dissections: genetic heterogeneity with a major locus mapping to 5q13-14. *Circulation.*, 103(20):2461-2468.

Guo, D. C., Papke, C. L., Tran-Fadulu, V., Regalado, E. S., Avidan, N., Johnson, R. J., Kim, D. H., Pannu, H., Willing, M. C., Sparks, E., Pyeritz, R. E., Singh, M. N., Dalman, R. L., Grotta, J. C., Marian, A. J., Boerwinkle, E. A., Frazier, L. Q., LeMaire, S. A., Coselli, J. S., Estrera, A. L., Safi, H. J., Veeraraghavan, S., Muzny, D. M., Wheeler, D. A., Willerson, J. T., Yu, R. K., Shete, S. S., Scherer, S. E., Raman, C. S., Buja, L. M., and Milewicz, D. M. (2009). Mutations in smooth muscle alpha-actin (ACTA2) cause coronary artery disease, stroke, and Moyamoya disease, along with thoracic aortic disease. *Am.J.Hum.Genet.*, 84(5):617-627.

Habashi, J. P., Judge, D. P., Holm, T. M., Cohn, R. D., Loeys, B. L., Cooper, T. K., Myers, L., Klein, E. C., Liu, G., Calvi, C., Podowski, M., Neptune,

E. R., Halushka, M. K., Bedja, D., Gabrielson, K., Rifkin, D. B., Carta, L., Ramirez, F., Huso, D. L., and Dietz, H. C. (2006). Losartan, an AT1 antagonist, prevents aortic aneurysm in a mouse model of Marfan syndrome. *Science.*, 312(5770):117-121.

Hahn, R. T., Roman, M. J., Mogtader, A. H., and Devereux, R. B. (1992). Association of aortic dilation with regurgitant, stenotic and functionally normal bicuspid aortic valves. *J.Am.Coll.Cardiol.*, 19(2):283-288.

Huntington, K., Hunter, A. G., and Chan, K. L. (1997). A prospective study to assess the frequency of familial clustering of congenital bicuspid aortic valve. *J.Am.Coll.Cardiol.*, 30(7):1809-1812.

Ikonomidis, J. S., Jones, J. A., Barbour, J. R., Stroud, R. E., Clark, L. L., Kaplan, B. S., Zeeshan, A., Bavaria, J. E., Gorman, J. H., III, Spinale, F. G., and Gorman, R. C. (2007). Expression of matrix metalloproteinases and endogenous inhibitors within ascending aortic aneurysms of patients with bicuspid or tricuspid aortic valves. *J.Thorac.Cardiovasc.Surg.*, 133(4):1028-1036.

Jackson, V., Olsson, T., Kurtovic, S., Folkersen, L., Paloschi, V., Wagsater, D., Franco-Cereceda, A., and Eriksson, P. (2012). Matrix metalloproteinase 14 and 19 expression is associated with thoracic aortic aneurysms. *J.Thorac.Cardiovasc.Surg.*, 144(2):459-466.

Kari, F. A., Fazel, S. S., Mitchell, R. S., Fischbein, M. P., and Miller, D. C. (2012). Bicuspid aortic valve configuration and aortopathy pattern might represent different pathophysiologic substrates. *J.Thorac.Cardiovasc.Surg.*, 144(2):516-517.

Koullias, G. J., Ravichandran, P., Korkolis, D. P., Rimm, D. L., and Elefteriades, J. A. (2004). Increased tissue microarray matrix metalloproteinase expression favors proteolysis in thoracic aortic aneurysms and dissections. *Ann.Thorac.Surg.*, 78(6):2106-2110.

Kroner, B. L., Tolunay, H. E., Basson, C. T., Pyeritz, R. E., Holmes, K. W., Maslen, C. L., Milewicz, D. M., LeMaire, S. A., Hendershot, T., svigne-Nickens, P., Devereux, R. B., Dietz, H. C., Song, H. K., Ringer, D., Mitchell, M., Weinsaft, J. W., Ravekes, W., Menashe, V., and Eagle, K. A. (2011). The National Registry of Genetically Triggered Thoracic Aortic Aneurysms and Cardiovascular Conditions (GenTAC): results from phase I and scientific opportunities in phase II. *Am.Heart J.*, 162(4):627-632.

Laforest, B., Andelfinger, G., and Nemer, M. (2011). Loss of Gata5 in mice leads to bicuspid aortic valve. *J.Clin.Invest.*,

Lee, T. C., Zhao, Y. D., Courtman, D. W., and Stewart, D. J. (2000). Abnormal aortic valve development in mice lacking endothelial nitric oxide synthase. *Circulation.*, 101(20):2345-2348.

Leeper, N. J., Raiesdana, A., Kojima, Y., Chun, H. J., Azuma, J., Maegdefessel, L., Kundu, R. K., Quertermous, T., Tsao, P. S., and Spin, J. M. (2011). MicroRNA-26a is a novel regulator of vascular smooth muscle cell function. *J.Cell Physiol.*, 226(4):1035-1043.

Lemaire, S. A., Wang, X., Wilks, J. A., Carter, S. A., Wen, S., Won, T., Leonardelli, D., Anand, G., Conklin, L. D., Wang, X. L., Thompson, R. W., and Coselli, J. S. (2005). Matrix metalloproteinases in ascending aortic aneurysms: bicuspid versus trileaflet aortic valves. *J.Surg.Res.*, 123(1):40-48.

Lichtenstein, E (1901). Zur Entstehung der Aortenaneurysmen, Dissertatio inauguralis. *Freiburg*

Lindsay, M. E. and Dietz, H. C. (2011). Lessons on the pathogenesis of aneurysm from heritable conditions. *Nature.*, 473(7347):308-316.

Lippe, B. (1991). Turner syndrome. *Endocrinol.Metab Clin.North Am.*, 20(1):121-152.

Loeys, B. L., Chen, J., Neptune, E. R., Judge, D. P., Podowski, M., Holm, T., Meyers, J., Leitch, C. C., Katsanis, N., Sharifi, N., Xu, F. L., Myers, L. A., Spevak, P. J., Cameron, D. E., De, Backer J., Hellemans, J., Chen, Y., Davis, E. C., Webb, C. L., Kress, W., Coucke, P., Rifkin, D. B., De Paepe, A. M., and Dietz, H. C. (2005). A syndrome of altered cardiovascular, craniofacial, neurocognitive and skeletal development caused by mutations in TGFBR1 or TGFBR2. *Nat.Genet.*, 37(3):275-281.

Loeys, B. L., Schwarze, U., Holm, T., Callewaert, B. L., Thomas, G. H., Pannu, H., De Backer, J. F., Oswald, G. L., Symoens, S., Manouvrier, S., Roberts, A. E., Faravelli, F., Greco, M. A., Pyeritz, R. E., Milewicz, D. M., Coucke, P. J., Cameron, D. E., Braverman, A. C., Byers, P. H., De Paepe, A. M., and Dietz, H. C. (2006). Aneurysm syndromes caused by mutations in the TGF-beta receptor. *N.Engl.J.Med.*, 355(8):788-798.

Macatee, T. L., Hammond, B. P., Arenkiel, B. R., Francis, L., Frank, D. U., and Moon, A. M. (2003). Ablation of specific expression domains reveals discrete functions of ectoderm- and endoderm-derived FGF8 during cardiovascular and pharyngeal development. *Development.*, 130(25):6361-6374.

Malfait, F., Coucke, P., Symoens, S., Loeys, B., Nuytinck, L., and De, Paepe A. (2005). The molecular basis of classic Ehlers-Danlos syndrome: a comprehensive study of biochemical and molecular findings in 48 unrelated patients. *Hum.Mutat.*, 25(1):28-37.

Malfait, F., Wenstrup, R., and De, Paepe A. (1993). Ehlers-Danlos Syndrome, Classic Type.

Malkoff, GM (1899). Über die Bedeutung der traumatischen Verletzungen der Arterien, die Entwicklung der wahren Aneurysmen und der Arteriosklerose. *Zieglers Beitraege* 25(2)

Matt, P. (2008). eComment: MMPs in gene- and protein-expression. *Interact.Cardiovasc.Thorac.Surg.*, 7(1):40-41.

Matt, P., Fu, Z., Carrel, T., Huso, D. L., Dirnhofer, S., Lefkovits, I., Zerkowski, H. R., and Van Eyk, J. E. (2007). Proteomic alterations in heat shock protein 27 and identification of phosphoproteins in ascending aortic aneurysm associated with bicuspid and tricuspid aortic valve. *J.Mol.Cell Cardiol.*, 43(6):792-801.

Matthias Bechtel, J. F., Noack, F., Sayk, F., Erasmi, A. W., Bartels, C., and Sievers, H. H. (2003). Histopathological grading of ascending aortic aneurysm: comparison of patients with bicuspid versus tricuspid aortic valve. *J.Heart Valve Dis.*, 12(1):54-59.

Mazzanti, L. and Cacciari, E. (1998). Congenital heart disease in patients with Turner's syndrome. Italian Study Group for Turner Syndrome (ISGTS). *J.Pediatr.*, 133(5):688-692.

Mendoza, D. D., Kochar, M., Devereux, R. B., Basson, C. T., Min, J. K., Holmes, K., Dietz, H. C., Milewicz, D. M., LeMaire, S. A., Pyeritz, R. E., Bavaria, J. E., Maslen, C. L., Song, H., Kroner, B. L., Eagle, K. A., and Weinsaft, J. W. (2011). Impact of image analysis methodology on diagnostic and surgical classification of patients with thoracic aortic aneurysms. *Ann.Thorac.Surg.*, 92(3):904-912.

Milewicz, D. M., Dietz, H. C., and Miller, D. C. (2005). Treatment of aortic disease in patients with Marfan syndrome. *Circulation.*, 111(11):e150-e157.

Milewicz, D. M., Guo, D. C., Tran-Fadulu, V., Lafont, A. L., Papke, C. L., Inamoto, S., Kwartler, C. S., and Pannu, H. (2008). Genetic basis of thoracic aortic aneurysms and dissections: focus on smooth muscle cell contractile dysfunction. *Annu.Rev.Genomics Hum.Genet.*, 9:283-302.

Miller, M. J., Geffner, M. E., Lippe, B. M., Itami, R. M., Kaplan, S. A., DiSessa, T. G., Isabel-Jones, J. B., and Friedman, W. F. (1983). Echocardiography reveals a high incidence of bicuspid aortic valve in Turner syndrome. *J.Pediatr.*, 102(1):47-50.

Mohamed, S. A., Aherrahrou, Z., Liptau, H., Erasmi, A. W., Hagemann, C., Wrobel, S., Borzym, K., Schunkert, H., Sievers, H. H., and Erdmann, J. (2006). Novel missense mutations (p.T596M and p.P1797H) in NOTCH1 in patients with bicuspid aortic valve. *Biochem.Biophys.Res.Commun.*, 345(4):1460-1465.

Mohamed, S. A., Hanke, T., Schlueter, C., Bullerdiek, J., and Sievers, H. H. (2005). Ubiquitin fusion degradation 1-like gene dysregulation in bicuspid aortic valve. *J Thorac Cardiovasc Surg.*, 130(6):1531-1536.

Mohamed, S. A., Misfeld, M., Hanke, T., Charitos, E. I., Bullerdiek, J., Belge, G., Kuehnel, W., and Sievers, H. H. (2010). Inhibition of caspase-3 differentially affects vascular smooth muscle cell apoptosis in the concave versus convex aortic sites in ascending aneurysms with a bicuspid aortic valve. *Ann.Anat.*, 192(3):145-150.

Mohamed, S. A., Noack, F., Schoellermann, K., Karluss, A., Radtke, A., Schult-Badusche, D., Radke, P. W., Wenzel, B. E., and Sievers, H. H. (2012a). Elevation of matrix metalloproteinases in different areas of ascending aortic aneurysms in patients with bicuspid and tricuspid aortic valves. *ScientificWorldJournal.*, 2012:806261

Mohamed, S. A., Radtke, A., Saraei, R., Bullerdiek, J., Sorani, H., Nimzyk, R., Karluss, A., Sievers, H. H., and Belge, G. (2012b). Locally different endothelial nitric oxide synthase protein levels in ascending aortic aneurysms of bicuspid and tricuspid aortic valve. *Cardiol.Res.Pract.*, 2012:165957

Mohamed, S. A. and Sievers, H. H. (2011). Ascending aneurysm in bicuspid aortic valve. In: Grundmann, R. Aortic aneurysm

Mohamed, S. A., Sievers, H. H., Hanke, T., Richardt, D., Schmidtke, C., Charitos, E. I., Belge, G., and Bullerdiek, J. (2009). Pathway analysis of differentially expressed genes in patients with acute aortic dissection. *Biomark.Insights.*, 4:81-90.

Nataatmadja, M., West, M., West, J., Summers, K., Walker, P., Nagata, M., and Watanabe, T. (2003). Abnormal extracellular matrix protein transport associated with increased apoptosis of vascular smooth muscle cells in marfan syndrome and bicuspid aortic valve thoracic aortic aneurysm. *Circulation.*, 108 Suppl 1:II329-II334.

Neptune, E. R., Frischmeyer, P. A., Arking, D. E., Myers, L., Bunton, T. E., Gayraud, B., Ramirez, F., Sakai, L. Y., and Dietz, H. C. (2003). Dysregulation of TGF-beta activation contributes to pathogenesis in Marfan syndrome. *Nat.Genet.*, 33(3):407-411.

Nesi, G., Anichini, C., Tozzini, S., Boddi, V., Calamai, G., and Gori, F. (2009). Pathology of the thoracic aorta: a morphologic review of 338 surgical specimens over a 7-year period. *Cardiovasc.Pathol.*, 18(3):134-139.

Nigam, V., Sievers, H. H., Jensen, B. C., Sier, H. A., Simpson, P. C., Srivastava, D., and Mohamed, S. A. (2010). Altered microRNAs in bicuspid aortic valve: a comparison between stenotic and insufficient valves. *J.Heart Valve Dis.*, 19(4):459-465.

Partsch, C. J., Pankau, R., Sippell, W. G., and Tolksdorf, M. (1994). Normal growth and normalization of hypergonadotropic hypogonadism in atypical Turner syndrome (45,X/46,XX/47,XXX). Correlation of body height with distribution of cell lines. *Eur.J.Pediatr.*, 153(6):451-455.

Pearson, G. D., Devereux, R., Loeys, B., Maslen, C., Milewicz, D., Pyeritz, R., Ramirez, F., Rifkin, D., Sakai, L., Svensson, L., Wessels, A., Van, Eyk J., and Dietz, H. C. (2008). Report of the National Heart, Lung, and Blood Institute and National Marfan Foundation Working Group on research in Marfan syndrome and related disorders. *Circulation.*, 118(7):785-791.

Pomianowski, P. and Elefteriades, J. A. (2013). The genetics and genomics of thoracic aortic disease. *Ann.Cardiothorac.Surg.*, 2(3):271-279.

Recklinghausen, FDv (1855). De pyaemiae theoriis.

Roberts, W. C. (1970). The congenitally bicuspid aortic valve. A study of 85 autopsy cases. *Am.J.Cardiol.*, 26(1):72-83.

Roberts, W. C., Vowels, T. J., Ko, J. M., Filardo, G., Hebeler, R. F., Jr., Henry, A. C., Matter, G. J., and Hamman, B. L. (2011). Comparison of the structure of the aortic valve and ascending aorta in adults having aortic valve replacement for aortic stenosis versus for pure aortic regurgitation and resection of the ascending aorta for aneurysm. *Circulation.*, 123(8):896-903.

Robinson, P. N., rteaga-Solis, E., Baldock, C., Collod-Beroud, G., Booms, P., De, Paepe A., Dietz, H. C., Guo, G., Handford, P. A., Judge, D. P., Kielty, C. M., Loeys, B., Milewicz, D. M., Ney, A., Ramirez, F., Reinhardt, D. P., Tiedemann, K., Whiteman, P., and Godfrey, M. (2006). The molecular genetics of Marfan syndrome and related disorders. *J.Med.Genet.*, 43(10):769-787.

Sakai, L. Y., Keene, D. R., and Engvall, E. (1986). Fibrillin, a new 350-kD glycoprotein, is a component of extracellular microfibrils. *J.Cell Biol.*, 103(6 Pt 1):2499-2509.

Schott, J. J., Benson, D. W., Basson, C. T., Pease, W., Silberbach, G. M., Moak, J. P., Maron, B. J., Seidman, C. E., and Seidman, J. G. (1998).

Congenital heart disease caused by mutations in the transcription factor NKX2-5. *Science.*, 281(5373):108-111.

Shi, X., Lu, Y., Wang, Y., Zhang, Y. A., Teng, Y., Han, W., Han, Z., Li, T., Chen, M., Liu, J., Fang, F., Dou, C., Ren, X., and Han, J. (2015). Heterozygous mutation of c.3521C>T in COL1A1 may cause mild osteogenesis imperfecta/Ehlers-Danlos syndrome in a Chinese family. *Intractable.Rare.Dis.Res.*, 4(1):49-53.

Swift, J., Ivanovska, I. L., Buxboim, A., Harada, T., Dingal, P. C., Pinter, J., Pajerowski, J. D., Spinler, K. R., Shin, J. W., Tewari, M., Rehfeldt, F., Speicher, D. W., and Discher, D. E. (2013). Nuclear lamin-A scales with tissue stiffness and enhances matrix-directed differentiation. *Science.*, 341(6149):1240104

Sybert, V. P. and McCauley, E. (2004). Turner's syndrome. *N.Engl.J.Med.*, 351(12):1227-1238.

ten, Dijke P. and Hill, C. S. (2004). New insights into TGF-beta-Smad signalling. *Trends Biochem.Sci.*, 29(5):265-273.

van, Rooij E. and Olson, E. N. (2007a). microRNAs put their signatures on the heart. *Physiol Genomics.*, 31(3):365-366.

van, Rooij E. and Olson, E. N. (2007b). MicroRNAs: powerful new regulators of heart disease and provocative therapeutic targets. *J.Clin.Invest.*, 117(9):2369-2376.

Ward, C. (2000). Clinical significance of the bicuspid aortic valve. *Heart.*, 83(1):81-85.

Wessels, M. W., Berger, R. M., Frohn-Mulder, I. M., Roos-Hesselink, J. W., Hoogeboom, J. J., Mancini, G. S., Bartelings, M. M., Krijger, R., Wladimiroff, J. W., Niermeijer, M. F., Grossfeld, P., and Willems, P. J. (2005). Autosomal dominant inheritance of left ventricular outflow tract obstruction. *Am.J.Med.Genet.A.*, 134A(2):171-179.

Wolpert (1905). Über die Häufigkeit und Entstehung des Aortenaneursmas, Dissertatio inauguralis. *Virchow Arch.*

Wooten, E. C., Iyer, L. K., Montefusco, M. C., Hedgepeth, A. K., Payne, D. D., Kapur, N. K., Housman, D. E., Mendelsohn, M. E., and Huggins, G. S. (2010). Application of gene network analysis techniques identifies AXIN1/PDIA2 and endoglin haplotypes associated with bicuspid aortic valve. *PLoS.One.*, 5(1):e8830

Index

A

B

C

D

E

F

G

H

I

N

O

P

T

U

V

W

X

Y